Family Emergencies

Betty Ann Falletta

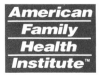

Medical Board

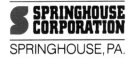

SPRINGHOUSE CORPORATION

SPRINGHOUSE, PA.

Program Director
Stanley Loeb

Clinical Director
Barbara McVan, RN

Clinical Editor
Donna Hilton, RN,
CCRN, CEN

Art Director
John Hubbard

Designer
Virginia Sloss

**Editorial Services
Supervisor**
David Moreau

Production Manager
Wilbur Davidson

The charter of the American Family Health Institute is to research and produce high-quality publications that enhance the health of individuals and their families. Essential to health are physical, emotional, and social well-being, not just the absence of illness or infirmity. The Institute's Medical Board has produced the *Health and Fitness* books to share up-to-date and authoritative information that can give readers greater personal control over their health maintenance.

Library of Congress Cataloging-in-
Publication Data
Falletta, Betty Ann, 1940-
    Family emergencies.
    Includes index.
    1. Emergency medicine—Popular works.
2. Medical Emergencies.   3. First aid in
illness and injury.   4. Medicine, Popular.
I. American Family Health Institute. Medical
Board.   II. Brunner, Lillian Sholtis.
III. Title.   [DNLM: 1. Emergencies—popular
works. 2. Medicine—popular works.
WB 120 F192f]
RC87.F34   1986   616.02´52
85-28346
ISBN 0-87434-018-7

The procedures and explanations given in this publication are based on research and consultation with medical and nursing authorities. To the best of our knowledge, these procedures and explanations reflect currently accepted medical practice; nevertheless, they can't be considered absolute and universal recommendations. For individual application, treatment suggestions must be considered in light of the individual's health, subject to a doctor's specific recommendations. The authors and the publisher disclaim responsibility for any adverse effects resulting directly or indirectly from the suggested procedures, from any undetected errors, or from the reader's misunderstanding of the text.

Contents

Family Emergencies

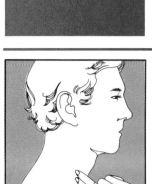

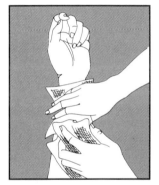

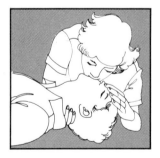

Introduction

The most important goals of first aid are keeping the victim alive, protecting the victim from any further injury, and getting medical help as soon as possible.

This book is designed to increase your preparedness, self-confidence, and effectiveness in an emergency. After reading this book, you should be better able to assess the severity of an emergency and to respond properly.

Think about the last medical emergency you experienced or witnessed. Was the situation life-threatening? Was the emergency the result of a sudden illness or an accident? If the emergency was accident-related, could the accident have been avoided? Did you give or receive first aid?

Accidents are by nature unexpected. Most are caused by carelessness, overconfidence, fatigue, emotional upset, failure to recognize safety hazards, and ignorance of safety rules. Because accidents don't "just happen" but are a result of human error, you can avoid most of them by learning and following a few simple safety rules.

Unfortunately, an accident may occur regardless of how careful you are. The possibility of an emergency situation is always present; without your quick action, permanent injury or even death can result. In an emergency, you may save a life by knowing what to do first, understanding why you are doing it, and then having the confidence to proceed.

First aid priorities

First aid refers to the immediate care you give to someone who has been injured or has suddenly become ill. Although all emergencies require immediate attention, you must first determine the nature of the emergency and then set priorities. The most important goals of first aid are keeping the victim alive, protecting the victim from any further injury, and getting medical help as soon as possible. Clear thinking and fast action will help you achieve these goals.

Follow up most first aid with medical attention

All life-threatening and many common emergencies require medical attention. Furthermore, some emergencies are best attended to at a hospital. When dealing with a life-threatening emergency or a serious common emergency, always try to get help without jeopardizing the victim. If other people are present, have one of them call a doctor or an ambulance while you administer first aid. While you wait for professional help, do whatever you can to help the victim.

While prompt attention to a serious emergency may save a life, the first aid you give is often no more than a temporary solution to a larger problem. The victim's future well-being may depend upon the professional evaluation and care that follows first aid.

Life-threatening and common emergencies

You must distinguish between life-threatening and common emergencies, because the causes and dangers in each instance are not always what they at first seem to be. What looks like a simple, uncomplicated emergency may be more life-threatening than an unpleasant-looking, but less-serious emergency.

If the emergency involves an accident that you have not witnessed, try to find out what happened before you do anything. Knowing the nature of the accident will help you avoid improper treatment in a life-threatening emergency. For example, you'd be taking a dangerous risk if, acting on your first impulse, you picked up an unconscious victim at the bottom of a flight of steps. You should first determine whether or not the victim is breathing and has a pulse. Then, find out if the person fainted or fell down the steps. The victim could have broken bones or a life-threatening head, neck, or spinal injury and should not be moved.

Follow this basic rule in all accident situations: Remove any danger from the victim, and move the victim only when his life will be endangered if he is not moved.

Like all emergencies, common emergencies require immediate attention. An abrasion, a broken ankle, a case of sunburn, a tension headache, or an animal bite are common emergencies, some of which are potentially more dangerous than others. Some common emergencies do not require professional medical attention, whereas others need immediate medical attention. The decision you make about an emergency will vary according to the circumstances that provoked the sudden illness or accident.

Rules of thumb for emergency action

Before doing anything else in an emergency, you should follow the ABCs of emergency care. You must check the victim's **Airway**, **Breathing**, and **Circulation**. Regardless of the injury, the victim will die if his airway is blocked and he cannot breathe, or if he loses too much blood. Think of the ABCs as the first things you deal with in an emergency, even if the victim complains about other parts of his body or if the victim's injury appears minor.

A is for airway

If the victim is unconscious, look for the rise and fall of his chest. Then, put your ear near his nose and mouth and listen for breathing. Feel for air moving in and out of his nose and mouth. Always look, listen, and feel for air movement. Also look and listen for symptoms such as noisy breathing, gurgling, or wheezing. If you don't hear or feel air movement, you must open the victim's airway before you can help him breathe. If a conscious person clutches his throat, can't cough, and can't speak, then his airway is obstructed. You must act immediately, or the choking victim will die. (See Choking, pp. 22-25.)

What you must do in an emergency

Look for the rise and fall of his chest, listen for breathing, and feel for air moving.

B is for breathing

When you are certain that the victim's airway is open, you should check his breathing. Look, listen, and feel again for air flow. If the victim isn't breathing, give artificial respiration. (See Artificial Respiration, pp. 20-21.)

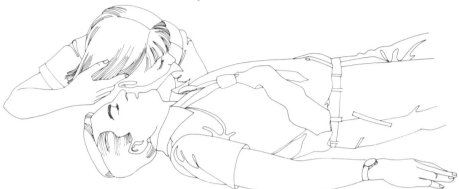

Look, listen, and feel again for air flow.

C is for circulation

Check the victim's pulse to find out if his heart is beating. If you can't feel a pulse in his wrist, check at the carotid artery in his neck alongside his Adam's apple. If you're sure you can't feel a pulse, use cardiopulmonary resuscitation. (See CPR, pp. 32-34.)

After you have followed the ABCs, summon medical help and stay with the victim until the doctor or ambulance arrives.

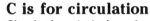

Check the victim's pulse.

When You're Alone and Need First Aid

1. Calm yourself.

When you take the time to learn first aid procedures, you'll be able to provide better emergency care for others and for yourself. If you are injured and alone, try to remain calm before you decide what action to take.

Procedures: Self-help

1. Calm yourself, and quickly evaluate the problem.
2. Follow the first-aid steps for your emergency situation. For example, you should be able to stop excess bleeding, bandage a sprain, and clean a wound.
3. Then ask yourself these questions: *Do I need help? Where is the nearest person? How can I get help?* If you need help, try to get it.
4. Don't overexert yourself.

2. Evaluate the problem.

3. Follow first aid steps.

4. Ask questions.

5. Don't overexert yourself.

What to Put in a First Aid Kit

You may save a life by knowing what to do first, understanding why you are doing it, and then having the confidence to proceed.

You don't have to spend a lot of money for a basic first aid kit. The kit should be labeled, portable, and easily accessible to adults, but out of a child's reach.

Include the following items in your first aid kit:

1. roll of adhesive tape (½-inch width)
2. sterile gauze dressings (2 and 4-inch squares)
3. roll of gauze bandage (4-inch width)
4. roll of elastic bandage and clips
5. adhesive strips of various sizes
6. cotton applicators
7. two triangular bandages
8. rubbing alcohol
9. safety pins
10. pair of blunt scissors
11. tweezers
12. eye cup
13. needle
14. aspirin or aspirin substitute
15. syrup of ipecac
16. thermometer
17. pencil and paper
18. tube of antibiotic ointment
19. eye pad

Safety in the Home

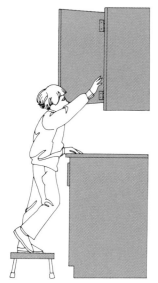

In the kitchen

1. Turn stove pot handles inward so that the pots can't be pulled to the floor or knocked over.
2. Wipe up spills immediately.
3. Install a safety gate with a childproof lock at the kitchen entrance, if you have small children.
4. Climb on a step stool, not on a counter, table, or chair to avoid falls.
5. Wear a cooking mitt and lift pot lids away from you to avoid steam burns.
6. Use a nonslip kitchen rug or put nonslip backing on your rug.
7. Close cabinet doors and drawers.
8. Don't reach into the toaster with utensils.
9. Lock cleaning materials, medicines, and poisons in cabinets, if you have small children.
10. Store sharp knives out of a child's reach.
11. Ventilate gas units.

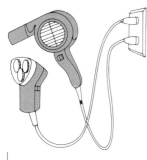

In the bathroom

12. Use a nonslip mat or strip in the bathtub.
13. Use a nonslip rug or washable wall-to-wall carpeting in the bathroom.
14. Make sure each electric appliance has its own socket.
15. Do not use an electric razor, hair dryer, radio, or other electric appliance when you are in contact with water.
16. Set the water heater at a temperature no higher than 120°.
17. Label all medicines and keep all prescriptions in their original bottles. Note expiration dates on prescriptions, and don't keep prescriptions that you no longer take.
18. Lock all medicines in cabinets, if you have small children.
19. Install handrails for the elderly near the toilet and bathtub.
20. Don't leave small children unattended in the bathtub or bathroom.

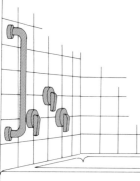

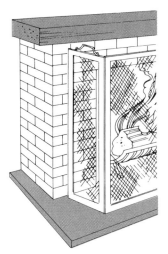

In hallways and on staircases

21. Light halls and staircases well.
22. Make sure staircase handrails are sturdy.
23. Fit staircase carpeting snugly.
24. Don't clutter staircases.
25. Install safety gates at the top and bottom of each staircase, if you have small children.
26. Install light switches at the top and bottom of each staircase.

In the bedroom

27. Have a light that you can reach from the bed.
28. Install metal guards on the windows in children's rooms
29. Don't wear loose-fitting slippers.
30. Install a smoke detector in each bedroom or at least one in the hallway outside the bedrooms.

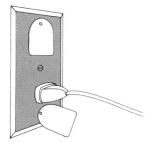

In the living room

31. Use a nonslip rug on a polished floor.
32. Mark or decorate glass doors.
33. Don't place objects on radiators or heaters.
34. Don't string cords where people walk.
35. Use a fire screen if you have a fireplace.
36. Put safety covers on unused electrical outlets.

In the garage or basement

37. Block the front and back wheels of your car before you work under it.
38. Keep all chemicals, tools, and appliances out of a child's reach.

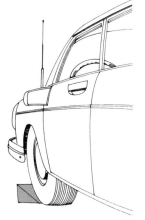

In the garden

39. Don't leave discarded or unused tools lying around.
40. Don't let unattended children play near pools and ponds.
41. Install fences, life belts, ropes, and poles if you have a swimming pool.
42. Don't use electric mowers in the rain or on wet grass.
43. Repair paths immediately, when necessary.
44. Use the correct tools for barbecuing.

What to Do at a Road Accident

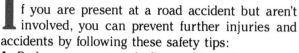

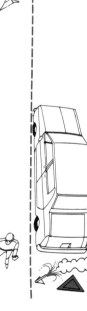

If you are present at a road accident but aren't involved, you can prevent further injuries and accidents by following these safety tips:

1. Park your car at a safe distance from the accident.
2. Warn oncoming traffic with a red reflecting signal, flashlight, or other device. (Do not light flares near gasoline.)
3. Switch off the engines of all vehicles involved in the accident.
4. Put out any fires with fire extinguishers.
5. Station available adults behind, and in front of, the wreckage to warn two-way traffic, especially on an undivided highway.

Attend to the injured by following these safety tips:

1. Get a message to emergency services. (Another motorist may take care of relaying the necessary information: the location of the accident, the number of people injured or trapped, the number of cars, whether a vehicle is burning.)
2. Don't move the injured unless his life is in danger.
3. Give first aid to those most in need. (Minor injuries can be treated later.)
4. Check each victim's airway and give necessary artificial respiration.
5. Control bleeding. (See Bleeding, pp. 14-18.)
6. Keep the victims comfortable.
7. Wait for emergency assistance.

If you have caused or been involved in an accident:

1. Stay at the accident scene for a reasonable time.
2. Give your name, address, the name of the owner of the vehicle, and the car registration number to the other driver or anyone who has good reason to ask for them.
3. Get the appropriate information from the other driver.
4. Have someone call the police and, if necessary, an ambulance.

Care of an Amputated Limb

A severed part of a person can sometimes be reattached. The proper care of a severed part from the time of the injury until it reaches the hospital may help prevent the victim from becoming disfigured or handicapped. The care and well-being of the victim, however, must always take precedence over care of the severed part. Call an ambulance or take the patient and the severed part to the hospital immediately.

Procedure: Care of an amputated limb

1. Do not put the part in water.

2. Wrap the part in a damp cloth and place a plastic bag over it.

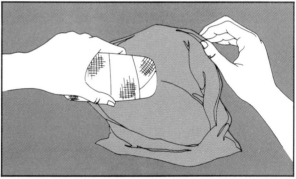

3. Fill a second plastic bag with ice cubes and place the bag containing the part inside the second bag.

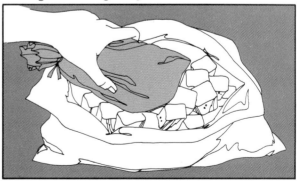

Bleeding

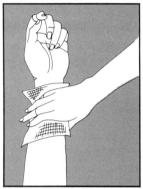

Direct pressure to the wound should stop bleeding.

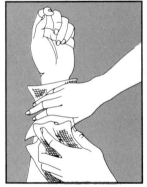

If bleeding continues, add more dressing while maintaining pressure on the wound.

A healthy human adult's circulatory system contains about 10 pints of blood. A small loss of blood produces no serious side effects; however, a blood loss of 2 or more pints is life-threatening.

External bleeding

At one time or another, we've all suffered a cut or scrape that has bled. External bleeding occurs when blood escapes from a wound in the skin. The blood can come from a vein, an artery, or a capillary.

Your most important goal when dealing with serious external bleeding is to stop the flow of blood so that a clot will form. Once formed, the clot blocks the blood flow from the damaged blood vessel, and bleeding stops. Your next order of business is to prevent infection and get the victim to the hospital for blood replacement (a transfusion) if the bleeding is severe.

Signs and symptoms: External bleeding

Bleeding from a vein is dark red, flows steadily, and can be very minor to very severe. Arterial bleeding looks bright red, is often profuse, and may spurt with each heartbeat. Bleeding from arteries is much less common than bleeding from veins. A minor scrape or shallow cut usually produces bleeding from capillaries, which is bright red, and usually oozes from the wound.

Procedure: External bleeding

1. Have someone call an ambulance.
2. Don't move the victim until you have treated the bleeding. You may find moving the victim necessary if he is in a dangerous location.
3. Apply direct pressure to the wound. Use a clean cloth, a large gauze pad, or your bare hand if no dressing is available. Press the wound directly for about 10 to 15 minutes. If the victim has a large, gaping wound, pinch the edge of the wound for about 3 minutes before applying pressure.
4. Don't remove the dressing if bleeding starts again. Apply additional dressing while maintaining the pressure to the wound.

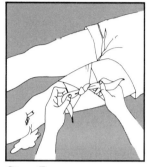

Step 7a

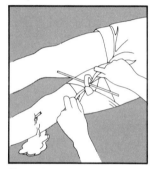

Step 7b

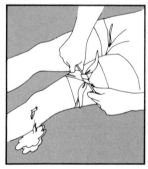

Step 7c

5. If you do not suspect a bone break and if the wound is in the arm or leg, raise the limb slowly. Try to keep the limb at a higher level than the heart.

6. If bleeding from the arm or leg doesn't stop with direct pressure, go a step further. Keeping one hand on the wound, use your free hand to apply pressure to the artery that is supplying blood to the wound by pressing it against the underlying bone. This procedure is known as the indirect pressure method. The different points that you press in the indirect pressure method are called pressure points (see the chart on page 16). Use the direct and indirect pressure methods at the same time and elevate the limb. Continue until the bleeding stops.

7. When you use a tourniquet, you may be sacrificing a limb to save a life. Once you use a tourniquet, take the victim to a hospital immediately.

Caution: Use a tourniquet only as a last resort.

a. Make the tourniquet from cloth folded to 2-inch width. Place it 2 inches above the edge of the wound, between the wound and the heart. Don't allow the tourniquet to touch the wound.

b. Wrap the tourniquet tightly around the limb twice and tie an overhand knot. Then place a stick or other similar object on the knot and tie another knot to hold the stick.

c. Slowly twist the stick to tighten the tourniquet only until the bleeding stops. Once the bleeding stops, do not twist the stick any further.

d. Secure the tourniquet with the loose ends of the material. Don't remove the tourniquet once you have used it.

e. Record the time the tourniquet was applied. For example, place a note in a prominent place on the victim's clothing. Be sure to tell the doctor or medical workers what time the tourniquet was applied.

8. When bleeding has stopped, bandage firmly.

9. Treat the victim for shock. (See Shock, pp. 38-43.)

Internal bleeding

Mr. Gina is thirsty and restless, and his skin is pale, wet, and cool. He has just coughed up a dark substance that has the color and texture of coffee grounds. Mr. Gina may be suffering from internal bleeding.

The signs that indicate internal bleeding are different from the signs that indicate external bleeding. The means used to control the two kinds of bleeding

Pressure points to control bleeding

If applying direct pressure doesn't stop the bleeding, then apply pressure to the artery that supplies blood to the wound. Use the pressure points shown.

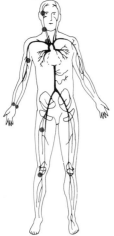

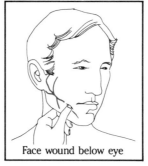
Face wound below eye

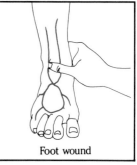
Foot wound

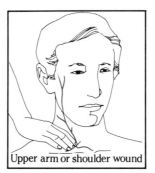
Upper arm or shoulder wound

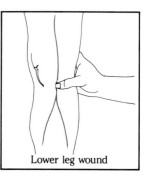
Lower leg wound

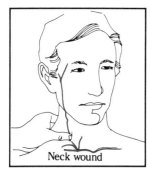
Neck wound

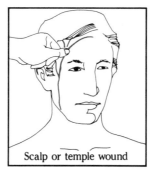
Scalp or temple wound

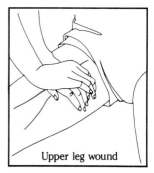
Upper leg wound

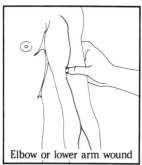
Elbow or lower arm wound

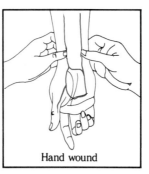
Hand wound

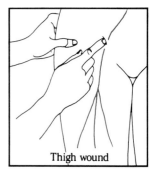
Thigh wound

The circulatory system

The human circulatory system consists of three main parts: the heart, the blood, and blood vessels. Your heart is a muscular pumping organ in your chest that keeps blood moving through your body.

Arteries are blood vessels that carry blood away from the heart. Arteries carry oxygen-rich blood from the left side of the heart to smaller and smaller arteries that reach all parts of your body. Nutrients and oxygen travel through your arteries to smaller vessels called capillaries, finally passing through the thin capillary walls into your body cells.

At the same time, cell wastes pass from the body cells to the capillaries through the capillary walls into the blood as it journeys back to the heart. Capillaries join large blood vessels called veins, which carry blood back to your heart's right side.

are also different. Blood that leaks into body cavities can't be stopped by pressure or by any of the procedures used to control external bleeding. You'll be of vital assistance to someone who's suffering from internal injuries and bleeding if you:

• learn to identify the types of injuries that could result in internal bleeding.

• learn to recognize the signs of internal bleeding.

• carefully observe the victim's condition.

Injuries that can cause internal bleeding

1. Any severe blow to the abdomen, chest, or head.
2. Broken bones and puncture wounds such as stabbing and bullet injuries, which may damage large blood vessels.

Caution: Sometimes, signs of internal bleeding may not show for hours or days after the injury.

Signs and symptoms: Internal bleeding

1. Bleeding from the ears, nose, or mouth may indicate a head injury. Nosebleeds and cuts in or on the mouth are not life-threatening emergencies.

2. Vomited or coughed blood may indicate chest or abdominal injury. Vomited blood that looks like coffee grounds could be from a stomach ulcer, whereas frothy, pale blood may be from a punctured lung.

3. A painful, tender abdomen that may become swollen and rigid.

4. Blood passed in urine and stools. A small amount of bright, red blood in the toilet bowl or on toilet tissue may be a sign of bleeding hemorrhoids; this isn't life-threatening, whereas heavy and rapid bleeding from the rectum may point to a serious disorder. Black or maroon-colored stools may indicate bleeding from the upper gastrointestinal tract.

The following symptoms of shock may indicate internal bleeding:

5. The victim will be thirsty, restless, and anxious.

6. The victim will be pale, wet, and cool.

7. The victim will feel weak.

8. The victim's pulse will be rapid and weak.

9. The victim's breathing will be fast, irregular, and shallow.

Procedure: Internal bleeding
Conscious victim

1. Have someone call an ambulance.
2. Have the victim lie down with his lower legs elevated. A victim of a chest injury should rest in a sitting position. Keep the victim warm.
3. Check and record the victim's pulse every five minutes.
4. Don't give the victim any fluids by mouth.

Unconscious victim

1. Have someone call an ambulance.
2. Place the victim on his side with his head also to the side. You can keep the victim's airway open by holding the jaw forward. Elevate his lower legs.
3. Keep the victim warm.
4. Check and record the victim's pulse every five minutes.
5. Don't give the victim any fluids by mouth.

Taking your pulse

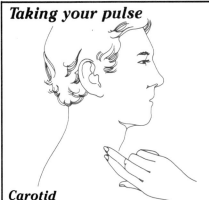

Carotid

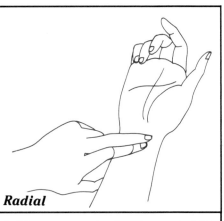

Radial

The pulse

If you place two fingers on the side of your neck next to your Adam's apple and press lightly, you'll feel a throb in an artery. This throb is known as your carotid pulse, and the artery you feel is the carotid artery. Hold your fingers on the inside of your wrist in line with your thumb. The throb you feel here is the radial pulse. The force of your blood pushing against the artery wall as your heart beats causes your pulse.

Procedure

1. Locate the radial or carotid pulse.
2. If you have a watch with a second hand, count the pulse for 30 seconds. Multiply your count by 2 to obtain the rate per minute.
3. Compare the rate to normal rates.

Normal pulse rates
- *Adult 60-100 per minute*
- *Child 75-110 per minute*
- *Toddler 80-130 per minute*
- *Infant 80-160 per minute*

Breathing

Respiration
Breathing, or respiration, begins when you inhale air into your lungs. Oxygen passes from your lungs into the blood circulating through your lung sacs. After your blood picks up fresh oxygen, it moves into your body, delivers the oxygen to your tissues, and removes waste products, such as carbon dioxide, from your tissues. The carbon dioxide passes out of your lungs as you exhale air.

Breathing involves stages of internal and external respiration. In internal respiration, your blood and tissues exchange oxygen and wastes. In external respiration, oxygen in your lung's air sacs passes into the blood while wastes pass from the blood into the air sacs. You then exhale the wastes out your nasal or throat passages and into the air.

Most people breathe without a second thought except when they have a cold or are breathless from overexertion or exercise. Anyone who has asthma, however, or who has choked on a piece of food may have wondered if they'd breathe again.

Some of the common causes of breathing failure are:
1. Choking
2. Drowning
3. Electric shock
4. Heart attack
5. Poisoning
6. Shock
7. Injury to lungs or chest.

When someone's natural breathing stops or becomes insufficient, you can help the victim breathe again by giving artificial respiration. During artificial respiration, you force air in and out of someone's lungs until the person's natural breathing starts again.

Signs and symptoms: Breathing failure
1. No visible or audible sign of breathing. Test the victim's breathing in three ways:
- **Look** for the rise and fall of the victim's chest.
- **Listen** for air flowing in and out of the victim's mouth or nose.
- **Feel** for exhaled air at the mouth or nose. Feel the chest wall for a sign of air movement.
2. Unconsciousness.
3. Blue lips, tongue, and nail beds. (This is not an indicator for dark-skinned people. If the victim is dark-skinned, check the mucous membranes, which will become paler.)
4. Dilated pupils.

Caution:
- **Do not give artificial respiration to someone who is breathing.**
- **When serious injury has occurred, you should first open the victim's airway, then concentrate on restoring breathing. (See #4 under Preparing victim for artificial respiration, on page 20.)**

Preparing victim for artificial respiration

1. If possible, place the victim on his back and loosen tight clothing.

2. If you suspect a back injury, do not move the victim. Give artificial respiration in the position that the victim is in.

3. Check the victim's mouth for anything that may be obstructing breathing, such as pieces of food, broken teeth, or dentures. If you see an object, remove it.

4. To open the airway, support the back of the victim's neck with one hand, place the other hand on the victim's forehead, and tilt the head backward slightly so that the nostrils are pointing upward. Another procedure for opening a victim's airway involves placing one hand on the victim's forehead and gently lifting the chin with the fingertips of your other hand. Be careful not to close the person's mouth completely.

Mouth-to-mouth procedure: Artificial respiration
Adult victim

1. Keep one hand behind the victim's neck, and use your other hand to pinch the victim's nostrils closed.

2. Form a tight seal with your mouth over the victim's mouth.

3. Quickly breathe into the victim's mouth four times without allowing the victim's lungs to deflate between breaths. (Fill your lungs completely between breaths.)

4. Maintain the head tilt, and look, listen, and feel for air movement.

5. If the victim still isn't breathing, form a tight seal with your mouth over the person's mouth, and breathe into his lungs.

6. Break contact with the victim's mouth and allow air to be released while you turn your head to watch the victim's chest fall. Keep the person's head tilted back and keep his nostrils pinched.

7. Take a deep breath and repeat the cycle. Breathe into the victim's mouth 12 times each minute.

8. Repeat steps until the victim is breathing regularly or until help arrives.

Adult mouth to mouth

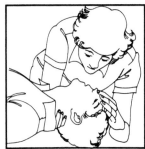

Step 1

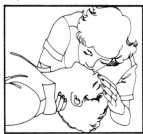

Step 3

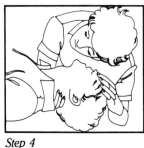

Step 4

Mouth-to-nose procedure: Artificial respiration Adult victim

1. Maintain the backward head-tilt position and with one hand under the victim's neck, use the other hand to cover the victim's mouth.
2. Seal your mouth tightly around the victim's nose and blow firmly into his nose, watching for the rise and fall of the person's chest.
3. Blow rapidly four times without allowing the victim's lungs to deflate between breaths.
4. Maintain the head tilt, and look, listen, and feel for air movement.
5. If the victim isn't breathing, form a tight seal around his nose and breathe into his lungs.
6. When allowing the patient to exhale, break contact with his nose and remove your hand from his mouth. Keep your other hand on his forehead.
7. Take a deep breath and repeat the cycle. Breathe 12 breaths each minute.
8. Repeat the steps until the victim is breathing regularly or until help arrives.

Infant mouth to mouth and nose

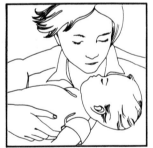

Step 1

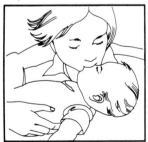

Steps 2 & 3

Mouth-to-nose procedure: Artificial respiration Infant victim

1. With the infant's back across your lap, tilt the head back slightly.
2. Place your mouth over the infant's mouth and nose.
3. With small puffs of air (one every 3 seconds) inflate the infant's lungs with enough air to make the chest rise.
4. To allow the infant to exhale, uncover both mouth and nose.

Choking

Why people choke
About 3,000 Americans choke to death each year. If you examine the closeness of the swallowing tube (esophagus) to the breathing tube (trachea), you'll understand how food easily travels down the wrong pipe.

The glottis lies just behind and below the tongue. Above the glottis is a flaplike structure called the epiglottis, which is attached to the root of the tongue. With normal swallowing, the glottis moves under the epiglottis so the flap of tissue seals off the trachea. This prevents the entrance of food or liquid into the trachea.

Mrs. Roth and her daughter Susan are having lunch to celebrate the young woman's acceptance into college. While they're eating, Mrs. Roth is suddenly unable to cough, speak, or breathe. She moves her hand to her throat—the universal choking sign. Fortunately, Susan knows what to do. Do you?

Not everyone has seen someone choking in public, but at some time in their lives many people probably have gotten a piece of food caught in their throats. Forceful coughing usually expels the food. If coughing does not clear the airway, other measures must be taken. Knowing some of the ways to help a choking victim can prove to be very valuable in an emergency.

Signs and symptoms: Choking
When a person is eating or a child is playing with a small object, the following may be signs of choking.
1. The victim grasps his or her throat.
2. The victim cannot speak.
3. The victim cannot cough.
4. The victim has difficulty breathing.
5. The victim begins to turn blue, pale, or ashen.
6. The victim falls unconscious.

Procedure: Choking
Conscious adult victim
1. Have someone call an ambulance.
2. Let the victim try to expel the food or object if he is able to speak or cough. This is the safest procedure. **Caution: If a person with the symptoms of choking can speak and is not choking, then the problem might be a heart attack.**
3. If the victim cannot speak and is having difficulty breathing, support the person with one arm, if possible. Then position the victim's head below his or her shoulders. Use the heel of your hand to give four rapid, forceful back blows over the victim's spine between the shoulder blades.
4. If the victim is lying down, roll the victim on his side so that his chest is against your knees. Then administer the four back blows the same way.

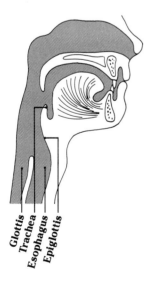

Glottis Trachea Esophagus Epiglottis

How to position your hands for the Heimlich maneuver

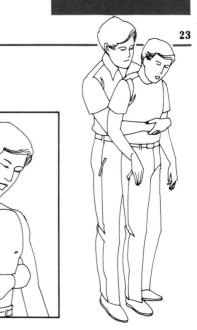

5. You'll need to use the Heimlich maneuver (abdominal thrusts) if the person continues to choke. To begin the Heimlich maneuver, wrap your arms around the person from the back, and make a tight fist with one hand, grasping it firmly with your other hand. Place your clasped fist, thumb in, against the victim's abdomen between the rib cage and navel. Don't tighten your arms. In a quick movement, press your clenched fists into the victim's abdomen at an angle toward your chin. Repeat four times if the first attempt is unsuccessful.

6. If the victim is lying down, place the victim on his back and kneel at his side, or straddle his hips. Then place the heel of one hand in the middle of the victim's abdomen, halfway between his navel and rib cage. Place your other hand on top of the first hand and interlock your fingers. Lean forward and press with a quick, sharp upward thrust four times.

Heimlich maneuver: Victim lying down

Preventing choking

Choking is a potentially life-threatening situation because the person who can't breathe has only minutes to live. The brain can't survive without air.

Some of the safety and etiquette rules that our parents taught us serve as excellent guidelines for preventing choking accidents:
* *Don't talk with a full mouth.*
* *Chew your food well.*
* *Don't put large pieces of food into your mouth.*

Pregnant or obese victim

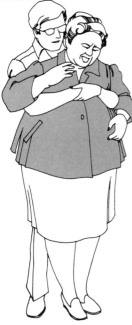

Use chest thrust on a pregnant woman or someone who's overweight.

7. If you see the food or object in the victim's mouth, remove it with your fingers.

8. Open the victim's airway and check for breathing after four back blows and four abdominal thrusts.

9. If you have no success with either method, repeat both methods until the object is expelled.

Unconscious adult victim

1. Have someone call an ambulance.
2. Place the victim on his back.
3. Open the victim's airway and attempt to restore breathing. (See Artificial Respiration, pp. 20-21.)
4. If you can't restore breathing with Artificial Respiration, turn the victim on his side facing you, and give four forceful back blows.
5. If you are still unsuccessful, roll the victim onto his back and give four abdominal thrusts.
6. Open the victim's mouth by pulling down his lower jaw and tongue. Look for the obstruction.
7. Repeat procedures 2 to 4 until medical assistance arrives.

Caution: All choking victims require medical assistance even if they start to breathe. The trapped object may have caused tissue damage.

Pregnant or obese victim Special considerations

1. Don't use the Heimlich maneuver (abdominal thrusts) on pregnant women or on obese people: Use the chest thrust instead.
2. When the victim is conscious and standing, move behind the person and wrap your arms around him, under his armpits.
3. Instead of placing your clasped fist against the top of the abdomen, place it on the middle of the breast bone and give four thrusts straight back toward you.
WARNING: Do not squeeze the victim with your arms.

*Helping yourself
when you're alone*

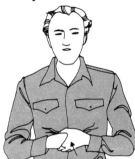

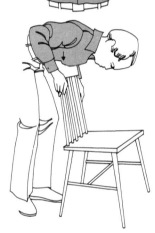

*What would you do if
you're alone and your airway becomes blocked?
Place the thumb side of
your fist into your abdo-
men, slightly above the navel and below the ribs.
Grasp your fist with the
other hand and press with
a quick upward thrust. Instead of your fists, you can
lean your abdomen against
the edge of a sink, table, or
chair, and press against it
applying pressure to the
same place in your abdo-
men.*

Infant or child victim

1. Have someone call an ambulance.
2. If the infant or child can breathe, cough, or cry, let
him try to expel the blocking object.
3. Give first aid if the infant or child has difficulty
breathing or coughing.
4. Place the infant or child face down across your lap
or forearm with his head down.
5. Use the heel of your hand to administer four quick
back blows between the shoulder blades. Naturally,
an infant or child should receive gentler blows than
an adult.
6. If the back blows don't dislodge the food or object,
turn the infant or child over and give four chest
thrusts. Place two fingers between the infant's nipples
and give quick, upward thrusts. If the victim is a
child, use the heel of one hand to deliver the chest
thrusts.
7. If choking continues, repeat back blows and chest
thrusts.

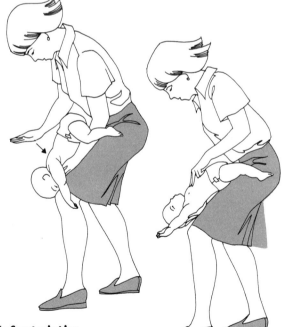

Infant victim
Give quick but gentle blows.

Diabetic Coma

If you find an unconscious person, first check for a bracelet or necklace that indentifies the person's condition. Then call an ambulance.

When a diabetic's system doesn't burn sugar at the normal rate, sugar builds up in his blood. Too much food, too little physical exercise, or too little insulin can cause a buildup of sugar in the blood. The excessive sugar buildup, which occurs over a period of several days, can lead to a diabetic coma.

Signs and symptoms: Diabetic coma

1. Restlessness and stupor, possible unconsciousness.
2. Weak and rapid pulse.
3. Vomiting is common.
4. Abdominal pain.
5. Victim's breath odor is fruity, similar to that of nail polish remover (acetone).
6. Deep, rapid breathing.
7. Dry, warm skin.

Procedure: Diabetic coma

1. Have someone call an ambulance.
2. Smell breath for acetone odor.
3. Look for an ID tag, often carried by diabetics.
4. Seek medical help immediately.

Medic Alert™ bracelet

Head, Neck, and Spine Injuries

The brain, the spinal cord, and the vast network of nerve cells throughout the body are part of a person's nervous system. The brain controls the nervous system. The brain collects, stores, coordinates, and remembers the messages brought to it by the sensory nerves. The spinal cord contains the nerve cells carrying messages to and from the brain. Thirty-one pairs of spinal nerves branch from the spinal cord.

Some parts of a person's body can regenerate themselves after extensive injury. Unfortunately, the major organs of the central nervous system, the brain and spinal cord, cannot regenerate themselves after they've been damaged.

If, for example, a person sustains a serious neck injury in a car accident, moving the person could cause paralysis and death. The victim should be moved only under certain conditions.

Head, neck, and back injuries are potentially life-threatening emergencies. Therefore, everyone should learn to use the appropriate first aid for an injury to the central nervous system or during the threat of such an injury.

Concussion and skull fracture

Susan hit her head on the windshield of her car in a head-on collision. Dazed and unconscious for a short while, she awakened with a headache, cold and clammy skin, and nausea. She didn't remember the details of the accident.

Susan's head X-rays revealed no break in the skull bones. She didn't have a skull fracture; however, she did have a concussion, a "shaking up" of the brain after an accident.

Gene, another passenger in the car, also hit his head. He, too, was unconscious for a short while. His pupils dilated, his temperature rose, his pulse slowed, and his muscles twitched and convulsed. Rather than a bump on his head, Gene had what looked like a dent. His X-rays revealed a broken bone that caused pressure on his brain. Gene had the type of skull

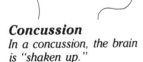

Concussion
In a concussion, the brain is "shaken up."

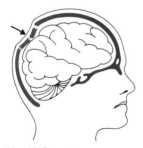

Skull fracture
In a skull fracture, a part of the skull presses on the brain.

Caution: Move the injured person only if the emergency is life-threatening, such as a fire or an explosion.

injury called a compression fracture.

Someone who becomes unconscious, even for a short time, after a blow to the head should see a doctor as soon as possible. The symptoms and signs of head injuries often don't appear immediately after an accident. Therefore, people should treat all head injuries as serious emergencies.

Signs and symptoms: Serious head injury

1. Headache, drowsiness, confusion, unconsciousness following a blow to the head.
2. A cut, bruise, bump, or dent on the scalp.
3. Inability to move the body (paralysis) or inability to move parts of the body (partial paralysis) after a blow to the head.
4. Loss of vision.
5. Bleeding from ear, nose, or mouth.
6. Blood-tinged fluid (cerebrospinal fluid) coming from the nose or mouth.
7. Vomiting.
8. Convulsions, which can be general or local, indicated by persistent twitching of muscles.
9. Loss of memory.
10. Disturbance of speech.
11. Unequal pupils.
12. Black eyes.

Jaw thrust without head tilt

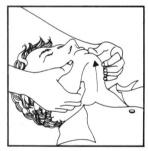

Opening the airway in a victim with a possible neck or spine injury.

Procedure: Serious head injury

1. Handle the victim carefully. Do not move the victim unnecessarily.
2. Have someone call an ambulance.
3. Keep the victim lying down.
4. If the victim isn't breathing and you suspect the possibility of a neck or spine injury, do not tilt the victim's head back. Instead, place yourself behind the victim's head. Grasp the victim's lower jaw by placing your thumbs on his jaw near the corner of his mouth, pointing your thumbs toward the victim's feet. With your fingertips at the angles of the victim's jaw, lift his lower jaw upward with your index fingers while pushing your thumbs down. This action causes the patient's jaw to jut forward without tilting his neck.
5. Restore the victim's breathing by giving artificial respiration if necessary.
6. Control bleeding from injuries and cover wounds. (See Bleeding, pp. 14-18.)

7. If normal breathing has been maintained and you do not suspect a neck or spine injury, in one motion, turn the victim's whole body to the side to allow secretions to drain and to prevent choking in case of vomiting.

8. Don't give the victim food or drink.

9. If you see that the victim's location is immediately dangerous to his life and that you must move the victim, do the following things before the move:

a. Immobilize and support the neck with a suitable collar. You can make a collar with fabric, folded newspaper, towels, or a blanket that has been folded to a width of about four inches.

b. Without obstructing the victim's breathing, fasten the collar and tie it loosely.

c. Support the shoulders and back.

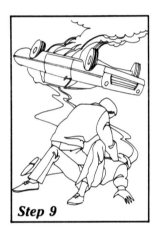

Step 9

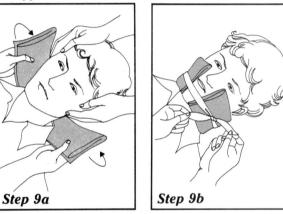

Step 9a

Step 9b

Signs and symptoms:
Neck or spine injury

1. Neck or back pain.

2. Numbness or tingling in the arms or legs.

3. Paralysis or partial paralysis, or weakness of arms or legs.

4. Disfigurement of the back or neck.

5. Painful movement of the arms or legs.

6. Tenderness along the back of the neck or spine.

7. Loss of bladder or bowel control.

8. Inability to breathe.

9. If victim is unconscious, presume that spine and neck injuries do exist.

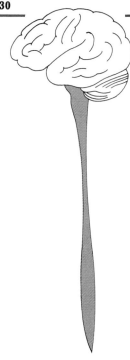

Procedure: Moving a victim with serious neck or spine injury

Remember: Move the injured person only if the emergency is life-threatening, such as a fire or an explosion.

1. Get a rigid support such as a board or door on which you'll carry the victim.

2. Four helpers are most suitable for the move, but you can manage the move with fewer people. Hold the victim's head in the alignment in which you found him. Don't let his head bend forward or backward. While holding the victim's head, have volunteers help you roll the victim on his side. Have someone place the board as close to the victim's side as possible. Then roll the victim onto the board, moving the victim's body as a unit.

3. If a board isn't available, don't lift the patient without six volunteers to keep his body in alignment.

The spinal cord
The human spinal cord is about two-thirds as long as the spinal column. Thirty-one pairs of spinal nerves branch off from the spinal cord. The spinal cord contains nerve cells that control motor reflexes and cells that carry messages to and from the brain.

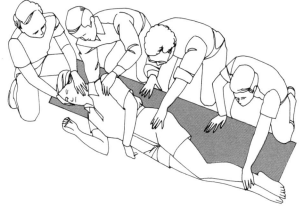

Moving the victim with his head, neck, and body aligned.

Heart Attack

Pain from other organs may seem like heart attack symptoms.

The heart, a muscular organ in the chest, pumps blood through the body. When adequate supplies of blood or oxygen fail to reach a part of the heart, a heart attack occurs. The lack of blood or oxygen may be caused by narrowed or clogged arteries. If the attack is severe, the victim may die suddenly.

The most likely candidates for a heart attack are middle-aged and elderly people who smoke, are overweight, and get little exercise. The pain of a heart attack is not necessarily sharp and immobilizing. In fact, a heart attack victim may overlook genuine heart attack symptoms because the symptoms don't seem life-threatening.

On the other hand, chest discomfort caused by other ailments may masquerade as heart attack symptoms. Chest pains can be caused by indigestion, ulcers, gastritis, gall bladder disease, pulmonary disorders, bruises, and shingles.

Signs and symptoms: Heart attack
1. Sudden crushing pain or pressure under the sternum, or a squeezing pain like a tight band around the chest. The pain continues.
2. Pain that extends to one or both shoulders and arms, or to the neck or jaw.
3. Weak or irregular pulse.
4. Shortness of breath.
5. Pale, clammy skin.
6. Weakness, especially with no cause such as exercise or strain.
7. Possible loss of consciousness.
8. Shock.
9. Bluish discoloration of the skin around the lips and in the nailbeds.
10. Nausea.

Procedure: Heart attack
1. Have someone call an ambulance.
2. Don't give the victim food or drink.
3. Place the victim in a partially reclining position, and loosen any tight clothing.

When a person isn't breathing and has no pulse, he'll die if you don't begin CPR. Even though it's an action of last resort, you'll need this procedure.

4. If you have been trained in cardiopulmonary resuscitation, and if the situation requires such action, administer it.

5. If the victim has a known history of heart disease, and requires medication that has been prescribed by a doctor (for example nitroglycerin tablets), let the victim take it.

Cardiopulmonary resuscitation (CPR)

CPR includes closed-chest heart massage as well as mouth-to-mouth respiration. Although CPR carries the risk of causing internal injuries such as a rib fracture or puncture of the lungs, stomach, or spleen, the procedure is worth trying if doing so can save a life. Of course, people trained by a paramedic or other professional can perform CPR with less risk of internal injury.

Procedure: CPR for an adult victim

(A person should use CPR when the victim isn't breathing and the heart has stopped.)

1. Give four quick lung inflations.

2. Locate the lower tip of the breastbone or sternum. Then measure up about two finger widths, and place the heel of your hand on this point.

3. Place one hand on top of the other and interlock your fingers to keep them off the victim's ribs. Keep ing your elbows straight, lean forward so that your hands and shoulders are in direct alignment and so that you can make full use of your body weight when you deliver downward compressions.

4. With the heel of your hands, apply steady, smooth pressure to depress the victim's sternum 1½ to 2 inches. Depressing the sternum forces blood from the heart's chambers. You should then relax pressure completely to allow the victim's heart to fill with blood. Don't lift your hands from the victim's chest when you release pressure, or you may lose the correct position.

5. Time your compressions at a rate of about 80 each minute. Count aloud to keep the compressions smooth and rhythmic. "One and, two and, three and..." After every 15 compressions, give two quick lung inflations without allowing the victim to exhale fully between breaths. (Actually, you'll be delivering about 60 compressions per minute because of the time lost while ventilating the victim.)

Details for giving cardiopulmonary resuscitation (CPR)

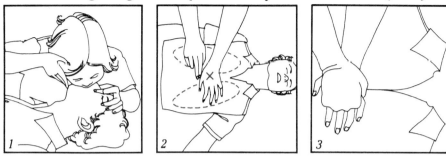

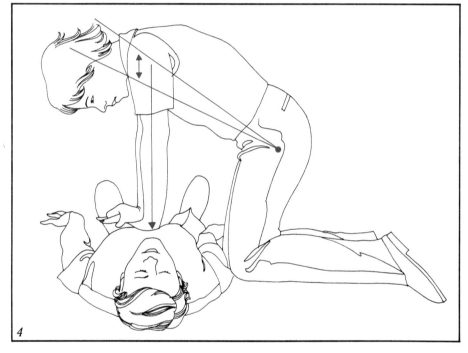

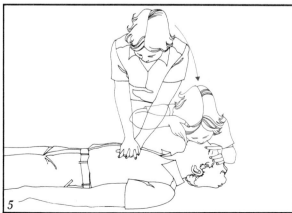

1. Give four quick lung inflations.
2. Locate the lower tip of the breastbone.
3. Place one hand on top of the other and interlock your fingers.
4. With the heel of your hand, apply smooth, steady pressure.
5. After every 15 compressions, give two quick lung inflations.

6. Check the victim's carotid pulse for 5 seconds after performing CPR for one minute. If you don't feel a pulse, give the victim two more ventilations and resume CPR.

Procedure: CPR for a child victim
1. Follow steps 1 to 4 above.
2. Time your compressions at a rate of 80 each minute. Give a lung inflation after every fifth compression.

Proper position for depressing an infant's sternum.

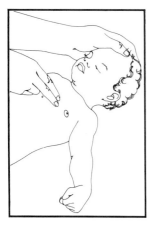

Procedure: CPR for an infant victim
1. Locate the victim's pulse inside the upper arm at the midpoint. (An infant's carotid pulse is hard to detect.)
2. Place the tips of your index and middle finger of one hand in the middle of the infant's chest, between the nipples. Deliver 100 compressions a minute, depressing the sternum ½ to 1 inch.
3. Give a lung inflation after every fifth compression.

Procedure: Two-rescuer CPR
1. Position yourself and the other rescuer on opposite sides of the victim, facing each other.
2. As your partner opens the victim's airway and tries to locate the carotid pulse, continue giving compressions.
3. If your partner feels a pulse, your compressions are adequate, but you should stop so that your partner can check to see if the victim's heart is beating on its own.
4. If no pulse is present, your partner should deliver one lung inflation, then tell you to continue chest compressions. Deliver approximately 60 compressions a minute while your partner delivers a full lung inflation on the upstroke of every fifth compression. Count out loud to maintain the right rhythm for two-rescuer CPR, "one-one thousand, two-one thousand, three-one thousand..." Your partner should check the victim's carotid pulse every few minutes.
5. You can switch positions with your partner if you get tired of giving chest compressions. When you want to switch, say "Change-one thousand, two-one thousand, three-one thousand..." On the fifth compression, your partner gives one lung inflation and moves into place for chest compressions. You move up to the victim's head and check for a pulse and breathing for 5 seconds. If you don't feel a pulse, inform your partner and continue CPR.

Poisoning

Poison symbol

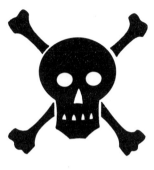

T wo-year old Kevin keeps himself busy all the time. He loves to empty drawers and cabinets to find out their contents. One day Kevin's mother finds him asleep on her bed with an empty bottle of pills next to him. Kevin may be the victim of poisoning.

Any substance that can harm or kill if inhaled, swallowed, absorbed through the skin, or injected into body tissues or the bloodstream qualifies as a poison. Prescribed medicines taken in the wrong dose, or by persons for whom the drug is not prescribed, can be poisonous. Most cases of poisoning happen by accident.

People can protect their families against poisoning by knowing the potential hazards in their households.

What to do if poisoning occurs
1. Know the signs of poisoning:
* *Abnormal behavior.*
* *Open container near victim.*
* *Difficult or abnormal breathing.*
* *Overstimulation or drowsiness.*
* *Unconsciousness.*
* *Burns on mouth or hands.*
* *Stains on clothing or around the victim's mouth.*
2. Keep the number of a Poison Control Center and nearby hospital emergency room near the phone.
3. Keep syrup of ipecac on hand.
4. Don't induce vomiting if a strong acid or alkali has been swallowed or if the victim is unconscious.

Signs and symptoms:
Poisoning by mouth
1. Open container near victim.
2. Abnormal behavior.
3. Unconsciousness.
4. Stains on clothing or around the victim's mouth.
5. Drowsiness or overstimulation.
6. Difficult or abnormal breathing.
7. Abnormal pulse rate.
8. Sweating.
9. Burns around the victim's mouth or on hands.
10. Unusual breath odors, body odors, or odors on the victim's clothing.
11. Dilated or constricted pupils.
12. Abdominal pain.
13. Nausea and vomiting.
14. Convulsions.

Procedure: Poisoning by mouth
Conscious victim
1. Have someone call an ambulance.
2. Call a Poison Control Center or the nearest hospital emergency room. Report:
* the age of the victim.
* the name or nature of the poison swallowed.
* the amount of poison that was swallowed.

Avoiding poisoning

Approximately 85% of the one million poisoning cases in the United States involve children. A child's tendency to put things in his mouth explains the numbers.
Many poisoning accidents can be prevented if you:
- *Lock all cabinets containing drugs, or keep drugs out of a child's reach some other way.*
- *Store all drugs in childproof containers.*
- *Discard leftover and outdated drugs.*
- *Never store hazardous substances in food containers.*
- *Use substances with hazardous fumes only when children aren't around and windows are open.*
- *Store household cleaning materials and toxic substances under lock and key or out of a child's reach.*
- *Never leave children unsupervised around dangerous substances.*

- when the poison was swallowed.
- the victim's symptoms, if any.

3. The victim may drink milk or water to dilute the poison. However, don't give milk to someone who has swallowed petroleum or gasoline or if the victim is having convulsions. Don't give fruit juice or lemon juice to any poison victim.

4. Follow the instruction of the Poison Control Center.

5. Substances such as acids and strong alkalis can cause serious damage if vomited. Petroleum products can escape into the lungs if vomited. Make sure you tell the poison control center if the victim swallowed these substances.

Caution: If the Poison Control Center recommends inducing vomiting, follow those instructions. The Poison Control Center may be preventing more harmful body effects.

6. Use syrup of ipecac to induce vomiting when its use is the suggested procedure. Give 2 tablespoons to an adult and 1 tablespoon to a child, along with a glass of water. Give a second dose in 15 minutes along with more water if the victim doesn't vomit.

7. When the victim vomits, keep his face down with the head lower than the body or his head tilted to the side so that he won't choke. Use a container to save the vomit.

8. Keep the victim comfortably warm.

9. Seek medical attention immediately. Take the poison container, leftover medication, and vomited material with you to the hospital.

Procedure: Poisoning by mouth Unconscious victim

1. Have someone call an ambulance.

2. Maintain an open airway and restore breathing, if necessary. (If the victim requires cardiopulmonary resuscitation, and you are trained, administer it.)

3. Call a Poison Control Center.

4. Don't give liquids to the victim.

5. Don't induce vomiting.

6. Loosen victim's tight clothing.

7. If victim vomits, turn his head face down or to the side so that the material drains out of the mouth and does not cause choking.

8. Seek medical attention immediately. Take poison container and vomit with you to the hospital.

Sources of poison
- *Cleaning fluids*
- *Insect repellants*
- *Furniture polish*
- *Plant food*
- *Gasoline, kerosene, and other petroleum products*
- *Cosmetics and hair preparations*
- *Paint and turpentine*
- *Bleaches*
- *Ammonia*
- *Poisonous plants such as mountain laurel and rhododendron*
- *Nonedible mushrooms*

Preventing poisoning by inhalation
1. Wear a mask to cover mouth and nose when spraying paints, insecticides, and other poisonous inhalants.
2. Open windows when you use poisonous sprays indoors.
3. Open the garage door before starting the car.
4. Don't light fires in enclosed areas.

Inhaled poison: Gas, smoke, or chemical fumes

Mrs. Frankel is working in her apartment, when she notices a faint smell of smoke. She checks to see that no fire is burning in her apartment; then she decides to check the hallway. In the hallway, she notices smoke coming from a neighbor's apartment. What is the first thing Mrs. Frankel should do?

Before you attempt to rescue someone who has inhaled smoke or poisonous gas, remember these points:

1. Call for help because you may need assistance.
2. Take several deep breaths of fresh air and then hold your breath before you enter the smoke- or gas-filled area.
3. Crawl or bend low in a smoke-filled room because you'll find more oxygen near the floor.
4. Keep your head above the fumes if automobile or other fumes are at ground level.
5. Take the victim away from the area to fresh air before attempting first aid.

Signs and symptoms: Inhaled poison
1. Unconsciousness.
2. Weakness or dizziness.
3. Headache.

Procedure: Inhaled poison
1. Take the victim to fresh air.
2. Check the victim's airway and maintain his breathing.
3. Give artificial respiration, if necessary.
4. Seek medical attention.
5. Check the victim for burns. (See Chemical Burns, page 62, and Eye Injuries, page 73.)
6. Keep the victim comfortably warm.
7. Loosen tight clothing.
8. Keep the victim in a reclining position until medical attention arrives.
9. If the victim is unconscious, place him on his side to keep his airway open.

Shock

In shock, a life-threatening emergency, the circulatory system fails to provide normal blood flow. To maintain an adequate blood supply to the brain, heart, and lungs, the body reduces the blood supply to the arms, legs, and skin.

Shock develops only in response to a serious illness or injury; however, the risk of shock exists with every medical emergency. Therefore, if you can identify a victim's emergency condition, you may be able to determine the victim's risk of going into shock and save his life.

Shock may be caused by such things as severe injuries, heart attack, serious bleeding, food or chemical poisoning, infection, broken bones, excessive loss of body fluids as a result of vomiting or diarrhea, and prolonged exposure to extreme heat or cold.

Eye changes in shock

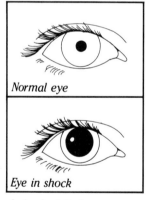

Normal eye

Eye in shock

A shock victim's eyes appear sunken and the pupils are dilated.

Early signs and symptoms: Shock
1. Restlessness, anxiety, and thirst.
2. Pale or bluish skin that is cold to the touch and possibly moist and clammy. Dark-skinned victims will have pale mucous membranes.
3. Weak, rapid pulse called "thready pulse", which is often too faint to feel at the radial artery but is perceptible in the carotid artery.
4. Rapid, shallow breathing, which may also be deep and irregular.
5. Weakness.
6. Nausea or vomiting.

Later signs and symptoms: Shock
1. Confusion and slurred speech.
2. Sunken eyes and dilated pupils.
3. Decreased body temperature.
4. Decreased blood pressure.
5. Mottled or blotchy skin.

Checklist for treating a shock victim:
- *Keep the victim lying down.*
- *Keep the victim warm.*
- *Check breathing.*
- *Treat injuries.*
- *Take the victim's pulse.*
- *Stay with the victim.*

Procedure: Shock

1. Have someone call an ambulance.
2. Treat the injury or condition first. For example, if the victim is choking, clear the airway and maintain breathing.
3. If you suspect a neck or head injury, do not move the victim.
4. If you don't suspect a neck or head injury, keep the victim lying down, preferably flat on his back.
5. If the victim is wounded on the jaw or lower part of the face, place him on his side so that fluids can drain from his mouth.

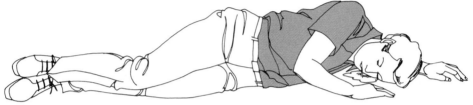

6. Open the victim's airway.
7. If injuries do not restrict the victim's position, elevate his feet 12 to 18 inches. Lower the feet if the elevated position increases the victim's pain or makes his breathing more difficult.

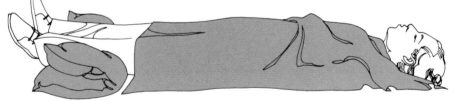

8. Keep the victim at a comfortable temperature, but not too warm.
9. Loosen any tight clothing the victim may be wearing.
10. Take the victim's pulse periodically.
11. Don't give fluids to an unconscious shock victim or when help is readily available.
12. If no medical help arrives for several hours and the patient is conscious, you may give lukewarm water with salt and baking soda. (Use 1 quart of water to 1 teaspoon of salt and ½ teaspoon of baking soda.) Give half a glass every 15 minutes to an adult victim. Give 2 ounces every 15 minutes to children ages 1 to 12 years, and 1 ounce every 15 minutes to infants 1 year or less.

How to treat an insect sting

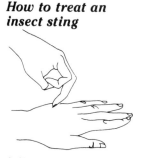

1. If a stinger is in the skin, remove it by scraping with a knife or fingernail.

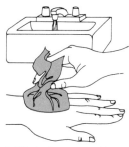

2. Wash the area with soap and water.

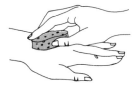

3. Apply cold compress or soothing lotion.
4. Keep the affected part lower than the heart.

Shock from reaction to an insect sting

The sting of a yellow jacket, a honeybee, a wasp, or a hornet can be very painful, and for some people the venom of these insects produces life-threatening consequences. Under normal circumstances, such a sting produces an intense burning sensation, redness, and itchiness followed by the appearance of a welt. Normally, a person can scrape out the bee's stinger, clean the area, and relieve the itchiness with cold compresses or an over-the-counter drug preparation.

However, people who are sensitive to the venom that accompanies an insect sting may experience a range of general (systemic) body reactions, including shock. For highly sensitive people, death can occur within 10 to 15 minutes after the sting. People who have a known sensitivity to insect stings should keep an emergency kit for stings available. Prompt action may save a life.

Signs and symptoms: Shock from an insect sting

1. Weakness or dizziness.
2. Abdominal pain or cramps.
3. Decreased blood pressure.
4. Collapse.
5. Unconsciousness.
6. Difficulty in breathing or swallowing.
7. Swelling in parts of the body—especially the feet, hands, and face (including the tongue).
8. Weak pulse.
9. Restlessness.
10. Hives.
11. Bluish color in the skin.
12. Nausea and vomiting.

Procedure: Shock from an insect sting

1. Have someone call an ambulance.
2. Open the victim's airway.
3. Maintain the victim's breathing.
4. In case of a bee sting, remove the stinger by scraping it with a knife blade or fingernail.
5. If the victim's life is at stake and no emergency kit is available, you should use a tourniquet to slow circulation around the sting. Use a tourniquet only if the sting has just occurred on an arm or leg.

Applying a tourniquet, Step 5a

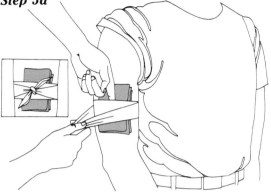

a. Tie a strip of cloth, cord, rubber, or a belt about 2 inches thick above the sting between the sting and the victim's heart. To avoid cutting off the victim's circulation, insert a finger underneath the band as you tie it.

b. Keep the affected part lower than the victim's heart.

c. Loosen the tourniquet every 5 minutes.

d. Use the tourniquet until medical help arrives.

6. If an emergency kit is available, have the victim administer an injection of epinephrine (adrenalin). If the victim is unable to do so, follow the victim's instructions or those in the kit.

7. Keep the victim lying down and comfortable.

8. Turn the victim's head to the side in case of vomiting.

9. Place an ice pack on the sting area to slow circulation and control swelling.

Electric shock

Reggie walks into the kitchen and finds that his mother has collapsed or fallen while ironing. The iron still in her hand, she lies unconscious. Reggie's mother is the victim of an electric shock. If Reggie knows how to proceed in an electric shock emergency, he will be able to protect himself and help his mother.

The sudden action of nerves and muscles in the body brought on by a discharge of electricity causes an electric shock. Electric shock results from direct contact with an electric current, and it can cause serious external and internal injuries or death. Common causes of electric shock include inadequate or faulty wiring, damaged appliances, and a lack of safety information.

Caution: Do not touch a victim who is in contact with electricity.

Signs and symptoms: Electric shock

1. The victim may be unconscious, and the victim's breathing may be poor or absent.
2. The victim may be in shock or in cardiac arrest.
3. The victim may have burns. With severe electric shock, the burns may look like explosive exit and entrance wounds, and the victim may have internal injuries.

Procedure: Electric shock

1. Move with extreme caution and turn off the power at its source or disconnect the power supply.
• *Do not* touch a victim who is in contact with electricity.
• Turning off the wall switch or the appliance will *not* remove the risk of electric shock.
2. If you can't turn off the power, remove the victim from contact with the current, but do not touch the victim yourself. If your hands are dry and if you're standing on a dry or shock-resistant surface, use a stick to push the victim clear of contact. You can also make a loop of rope and pull the victim away from the source of the current.

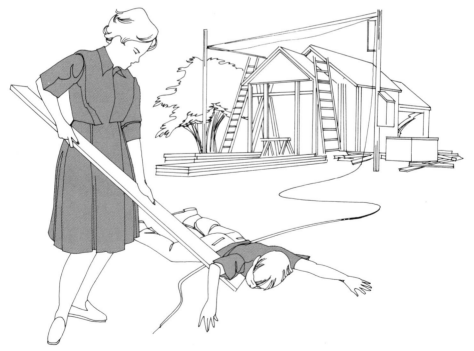

Using a board to move an electric shock victim.

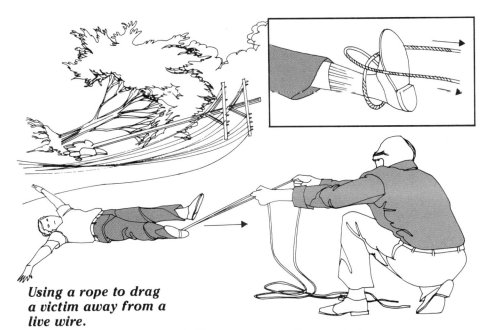

Using a rope to drag a victim away from a live wire.

3. Have someone call an ambulance.

4. If you can safely touch the victim, check his breathing. Give artificial respiration, if necessary.

5. If the victim also needs cardiopulmonary resuscitation, a combination of artificial respiration and cardiac compression, a trained person should administer the aid.

6. Treat the victim for shock if necessary, or prevent shock.

7. Treat burns and other injuries that may have been caused by a fall. All electrical burns are third degree, and you should treat them as such. (See Burns, pp. 60-62.)

   a. Do not immerse burns larger than 2 inches in cold or ice water, because the temperature change could cause circulatory failure, another life-threatening emergency. (See p. 38).

   b. Place a loose dressing over a large burn.

   c. Check the victim's skin for exit and entrance burns caused by electric current. Electric current may produce a whitish yellow entrance wound that looks charred or dented. Exit wounds from electric current may be small, may look like the entrance wound, or may look like explosive injuries.

Emergency procedure for serious burns

• *Get medical help immediately.*

• *Do not break blisters.*

• *Do not use creams, grease, or lotion on the burn.*

• *Treat the victim for shock. Keep the victim lying down, at rest, and comfortably warm. Elevate the victim's feet.*

The effects of electric current inside the human body

A person injured by an electric shock or lightning usually has internal damage. You may see burn marks where the electricity entered and left the body, but you won't be able to see most of the damage. This picture shows which internal organs or parts may have been affected.

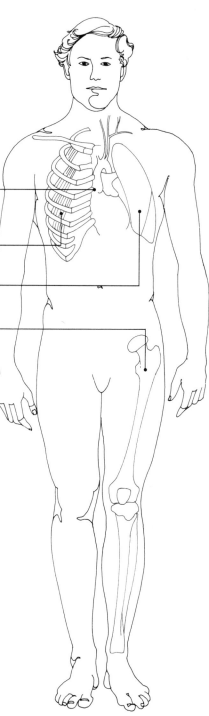

Heart ——————————
Beat is interrupted or may stop.

Muscles around the ribs ——————
Spasms interfere with breathing.

Lungs ——————————
Breathing may stop or fluid may collect.

Bones ——————————
May be knocked out of position or broken.

Caution: The size of the burn does not indicate if the injuries inside are serious. Get medical help immediately.

Insulin shock

Lena, an overweight diabetic, has decided to start an exercise program. For several days, she has jogged for a half hour before going to work. She has continued to take her insulin at the usual time and has not consulted her doctor about her exercise program. This morning she experienced muscle tremors while sitting at her desk. Then she felt dizzy and passed out. The company doctor diagnosed the condition as insulin shock.

Insulin shock is a low-blood sugar, or hypoglycemic, reaction to too much insulin. Skipped meals, an overdose of insulin, excessive physical activity, and emotional upset can bring on insulin shock. Unlike a diabetic coma, insulin shock occurs suddenly.

Signs and symptoms: Insulin shock

1. Dizziness, headache, or drowsiness.
2. Cold, clammy skin, with ashen color.
3. Rapid pulse.
4. Muscle tremors.
5. Excessive emotional reactions (crying or laughing) or excited behavior.
6. Convulsions.
7. Extreme hunger.
8. Unconsciousness.

Procedure: Insulin shock

1. Have someone call an ambulance.
2. If the victim is unconscious or in shock, don't give the victim food or liquids.
3. Give a conscious victim some form of sugar, such as candy, orange juice, or soda, in small amounts at a time.

Abdominal Pain

The abdominal cavity
The organs of your digestive system are located in the abdominal cavity. (A woman's reproductive system is also situated there.)

The digestive system breaks down the food you eat so that the body can absorb nutrients and eliminate waste products.

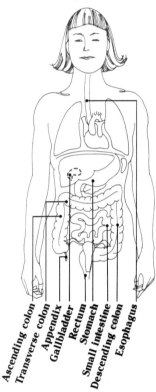

Ascending colon
Transverse colon
Appendix
Gallbladder
Rectum
Stomach
Small intestine
Descending colon
Esophagus

A s Cleo described her stomachache to Dr. Kalman, she pointed to the right side of her lower abdomen. Like many people, Cleo refers to any pain in the region from her rib cage down to her lower pelvis as stomach pain; however, the malfunctioning of any organ in the abdominal cavity can cause varying degrees of abdominal discomfort. The following guidelines can help a person decide whether or not to call a doctor.

Warning signals: Abdominal pain
Call a doctor if the victim:
1. Has pain that comes on suddenly or has continuous pain accompanied by fever and abdominal tenderness.
2. Has abdominal pain accompanied by backache and frequent urination.
3. Has had abdominal surgery.
4. Has an attack of vomiting or diarrhea that lasts for more than a few hours.
5. Has a recurrent pain in the middle of the abdominal cavity that is relieved by eating.
6. Is short of breath, weak, nauseated, pale and sweaty, and has pain in the upper abdomen.

Appendicitis
The appendix is a narrow, hollow tube (closed at one end) that is attached to the large bowel on the lower abdomen's right side. An inflamed, infected appendix results in appendicitis.

Signs and symptoms: Appendicitis
1. The victim experiences intermittent pain that starts anywhere in the abdomen and moves to the lower right abdomen. Pain may become constant.
2. The victim may vomit, have slight fever, or experience tenderness in the abdomen.

Procedure: Appendicitis
1. Call a doctor immediately or take the victim to a nearby hospital emergency room. Delay increases the danger of the appendix bursting.
2. Don't give the victim food or water.

3. Don't give the victim a laxative or an enema.
4. Don't apply heat to the victim's abdomen.
5. Place an ice pack on the area to give the victim some relief from pain.

How to avoid food poisoning

When you buy canned food, don't buy cans if they have:
* *rust spots*
* *dents or*
* *swellings.*

When you use home-canned foods, don't use a can if the
* *lid is bulging*
* *seal isn't tight*
* *color or odor is bad*
* *food contains molds or other growths.*

Carefully throw away any spoiled food so that children and animals can't reach it.

Food poisoning

If several people experience abdominal pain, nausea, headache, vomiting, and diarrhea after eating a picnic or other meal together, they may be suffering from food poisoning by staphylococci, one of the four major types of bacteria responsible for contaminated food. Most likely, the cold cuts along with the salads and desserts prepared with dairy products were not kept at a cool temperature. Food poisoning from staphylococci rarely causes death.

Botulism, on the other hand, is a lethal form of food poisoning. Home-canned vegetables, especially those with low acid content, can cause botulism if the vegetables were not washed or canned properly.

Signs and symptoms: Food poisoning

1. Abdominal cramps.
2. Nausea and vomiting.
3. Headache.
4. Diarrhea.

Additional signs and symptoms: Botulism

1. Sore throat, weakness, vomiting, and diarrhea.
2. Dimness of vision, drooping eyelids, followed by double vision.
3. Difficulty swallowing and talking.

Procedure: Food poisoning

1. Seek medical attention immediately if you suspect botulism. The victim must receive an antitoxin as soon as possible. Persons who are not yet ill but who have eaten foods suspected of being contaminated may also take the antitoxin.
2. Don't give the victim any antidiarrheal medicines such as Kaopectate.
3. Make the victim as comfortable as possible.
4. When vomiting subsides, or if it hasn't occurred, give the victim liquids in small sips to replace lost fluid.
5. Withhold solid food until the attack is over. Then, reintroduce the victim to bland solid food such as toast.

Allergic Reactions

Asthma attacks may be relieved by moisture.

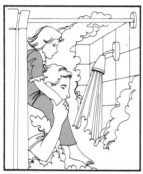

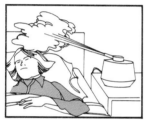

Asthma attacks may be relieved if the arms are braced to assist with breathing.

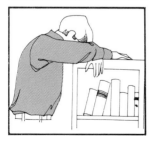

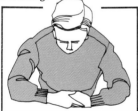

People who sneeze and have watery eyes in the springtime or break out in a rash every time they eat chocolate are experiencing an allergic reaction. Their bodies are reacting abnormally to usually harmless substances. Most allergic reactions, such as hay fever and hives, are not serious; however, some allergic reactions can be life-threatening emergencies. For example, if someone who is allergic to penicillin starts an antibiotic prescription containing the drug, the person's mouth and tongue may swell and block the airway.

Allergic asthma
Asthma, an allergic reaction, makes a victim's breathing difficult by causing spasms of the small breathing tubes, or bronchioles.

Signs and symptoms: Allergic asthma
1. Breathing difficulty, especially when exhaling.
2. A wheezing sound during breathing.
3. Faster than normal heart rate.
4. Heavy perspiration.

Procedure: Allergic asthma
1. Help the victim take his prescribed medication if he has seen a doctor for the condition.
2. Keep the victim calm.
3. Have the victim sit up.
4. Provide moist air for the victim to breathe.
5. Have the victim see a doctor if the condition has not been diagnosed, does not improve within a half hour, or if the condition worsens.
6. Have the victim brace his arms so that chest and arms can assist in breathing.

Back Strain

How to prevent back strain

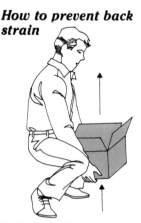

• *When you lift any object, do not bend stiff-legged. Bend your knees, use your thigh muscles, and crouch with your back straight.*
• *Use two arms to pick up a heavy object.*

Timothy is a construction worker in good physical shape. He exercises regularly and watches his weight. He has good posture and strong abdominal muscles. Despite his excellent physical condition, Timothy experiences a severe pain in his lower back. What could possibly be causing Timothy's back pain?

Low back pain triggered by a fall or by lifting a heavy object is fairly common among laborers like Timothy. Tension, arthritis, and poor posture also commonly cause low back pain.

Signs and symptoms: Back strain
1. Stiffness.
2. Aching with or without movement.
3. Muscle spasms.
4. Impaired function.

Procedure: Back strain
1. Have the victim apply a moist (heat) heating pad to the injured area.
2. Have the victim rest on a hard bed or other hard surface.
3. If the victim can tolerate aspirin, let him take two aspirin every 4 hours.
4. Apply hot compresses to the injured area or have the victim soak in a warm bath as many times a day as necessary until the pain diminishes.
5. Massage the victim's back.
6. If the pain persists, have the victim consult a doctor.
WARNING SIGNAL: Back pain between the shoulder blades or a shooting pain down either or both arms may indicate a heart attack.

Strengthening your back

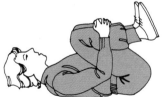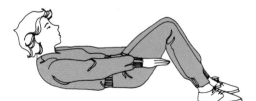

• *Strengthen your stomach to improve your lower back strength.*

Bites and Stings

Although exotic pets and strange animals do bite people, most bites and stings are inflicted by common insects and household pets known to the victims.

Animal bites

Animal bites can cause severe bleeding, tissue damage, and infection, and people should treat the bites as serious injuries. Wounds of the face, head, and neck are more dangerous than bites on other parts of the body. Even when an animal shows no sign of rabies, a doctor may prescribe rabies treatment for a serious bite. Any person bitten by an animal should get medical advice or care.

Caring for an animal bite

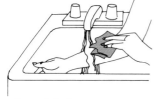

Steps 3 & 4

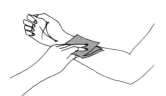

Step 5

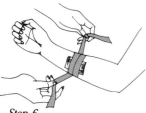

Step 6

Procedure: Animal bites

1. If the bite causes life-threatening bleeding to the victim, control the bleeding first. (See Bleeding, p. 14.)
2. If a domestic animal has bitten the victim, get the owner's name and address and find out if the animal has had a rabies vaccination.
3. Wash the bite thoroughly with soap and water.
4. Continue to flush the wound for 5 minutes with water.
5. Pat the wound dry with a sterile pad.
6. Cover the wound with a sterile gauze pad.
7. Call a doctor to find out if the victim needs a tetanus shot and rabies vaccination. (Adults need a tetanus booster every 5 to 10 years.) Dogs, cats, squirrels, raccoons, foxes, and other warm-blooded animals can carry rabies.

Snakebites

Most snakes in the United States are nonpoisonous. Two types of poisonous snakes, pit vipers and coral snakes, do exist in the U.S. Pit vipers include rattlesnakes, copperheads, and water moccasins. These snakes are called pit vipers because of the poison sacs, or pits, between their eyes and nostrils. Unlike pit vipers, the other type of poisonous snakes, coral snakes, rarely strikes unless provoked.

Most snakes are not poisonous, but you should have all snake bites checked by a doctor.

People who hike in an area where snakes may live, should wear high boots, long sleeves, and long pants. They should walk or climb where they can see clearly around themselves, use a walking stick if moving through high grass, step onto fallen trees rather than over them, and never put their hands into hidden places, such as crevices. In fact, most snakes are afraid of people; they will crawl away if given the chance. If bitten, a person must get help and antivenin.

Procedure: Snakebites

1. Have the victim lie down and keep him from moving.
2. Maintain an open airway and restore breathing, if necessary.
3. Keep the victim warm and calm.
4. Have the victim keep the bite immobilized and lower than his heart, if possible.
5. If you can take the victim to the hospital within 4 to 5 hours and if no symptoms develop, you do not have to provide additional first aid.
6. If mild to moderate symptoms develop, make a band (tourniquet) with a folded bandage, belt, tie, or other suitable material that is ¾ to 1½ inches wide.
• Tie the band about 2 to 4 inches above the bite, between the bite and the heart. Do not make the band tight. It should be loose enough for a finger to fit underneath. (Do not use a band if the bite is on the neck, head, or torso, and do not tie a band around a joint.)
• Check the tourniquet regularly, but do not remove it. Loosen the band if it becomes too tight.
7. Treat the victim for shock, and give artificial respiration or CPR, if necessary.
8. Clean the bitten area with soap and water.
9. If you have a snakebite emergency kit, use the blade in the kit. Make a ⅛ inch deep cut into each fang mark, making the cut ½ inch long. Use the suction cups in the emergency kit to remove the venom.
10. If you don't have an emergency kit, keep the victim calm, immobilize the part, and keep that body part lower than the victim's heart.
11. Treat the victim for shock, and give artificial respiration or CPR, if necessary.
12. Get to a hospital immediately.

Snakebites

This chart gives you information at a glance about four poisonous snakes—copperheads, cotton mouths, rattlesnakes, and coral snakes.

Name	Type of bite marks	Symptoms
Copperhead (Also known as pilot, adder) Copper colored head and markings.	Fang and teeth marks.	• Severe pain. • Rapid swelling at the bite. • Skin discoloration around the bite. • Possible weakness, nausea, dimness of vision, and fever. • Possible breathing difficulty, shock, and rapid heartbeat
Cotton mouth (Also known as water moccasin) Has slitlike eyes	Same as above	Same as above
Rattlesnake Has rattles on the end of its tail.	Same as above	Same as above
Coral snake Has red, yellow, and black rings.	Teeth marks. May or may not have fang marks.	• Slight burning pain. • Mild swelling. • Other symptoms may develop after several hours and may progress rapidly. • Possible sweating, nausea, vomiting, and weakness. • Blurred vision and droopy eyelids. • Difficulty breathing and speaking. • Possible shock and paralysis.

Insect bites

This chart gives you information at a glance about three poisonous insects—black widow spiders, brown recluse spiders, and scorpions.

Name and appearance	Symptoms
Black widow spider Shiny black body with a red or yellow hour-glass marking on its underside.	• Local swelling with tiny red bite marks. • Severe stinging pain initially, then dull numbing pain. • Painful cramps of abdominal and other muscles. • Possible restlessness, dizziness, nausea, headache, vomiting, shock, profuse sweating, convulsions, and respiratory depression.
Brown recluse spider (Also called fiddler spider) Tan or yellow body with a violin shaped marking on its back.	• Stinging sensation. • Redness. • Mild or no pain with bite; pain increases over 8 hour period. • Over the next 48 hours: possible chills, fever, nausea, vomiting, and joint pain. • Formation of an open sore within 2 to 3 weeks.
Scorpion Resembles a miniature lobster.	• Severe burning pain at the site of the sting. • Local swelling and tenderness. • Abdominal pain. • Within 1 to 3 hours: itchy eyes, mouth, and throat, impaired speech, drowsiness, nausea, and vomiting. • Possible breathing difficulty and heart failure. • Signs and symptoms last 1 to 3 days.

Procedure: Poisonous insects

1. Maintain an open airway and restore breathing, if necessary.
2. Keep the bitten area lower than the rest of the body, if possible.
3. Keep the victim warm and quiet.
4. Cleanse the bite and surrounding areas.
5. Apply cold compresses or ice to the bite.
6. Seek medical attention immediately.

Sea creatures

This chart gives you information at a glance about two poisonous sea creatures—jellyfish and stingrays.

Name and appearance	Symptoms
Jellyfish Disklike with tentacles.	• Severe burning pain. • Redness in the area of contact. • Skin rash. • Possible nausea, vomiting, diarrhea, convulsions, muscle cramps, shock, and breathing difficulty.
Stingray Flat, sharklike fish with tough skin and a tail with a sharp spine.	• Laceration or puncture wound. • Possible nausea, vomiting, diarrhea, muscle cramps, convulsions, and breathing difficulty.

Procedure: Poisonous sea animals

1. For jellyfish, use a towel to gently wipe away tentacles. Then wash the area with rubbing alcohol or a dilute solution of ammonia. Treat the victim for shock, if necessary. Call a doctor.

2. For stingrays, control bleeding. Then soak the bitten area in hot water. Treat the victim for shock. Check the victim's breathing, and be prepared to give artificial respiration or CPR. Get medical attention for cleansing the wound and for removal of spine fragments.

Human bites

An open wound or a puncture wound caused by human teeth breaking the skin requires immediate attention. In fact, a person's mouth is more heavily contaminated with bacteria than an animal's mouth, causing a higher risk of infection.

Procedure: Human bites

1. Control severe bleeding.
2. Cleanse the wound thoroughly with soap and water.
3. Cover the wound.
4. See a doctor immediately.

Bone Injuries

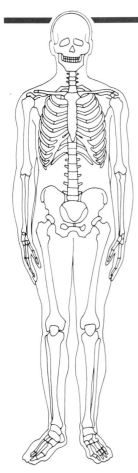

While playing ball with her friends, Helena fell and landed on her knees with her arms outstretched. After she fell, Helena went home because her wrist was painful, tender, bruised, and swollen, and she didn't have much strength in her arm. What injuries could Helena have sustained in her fall? Did she do something wrong? In her fall, Helena may have broken several bones.

A break or crack in a bone is called a fracture. When parts of the broken bone cut through the skin, the break is called an open fracture. When the skin is not broken over a fracture, the fracture is called closed.

Some bone breaks are obvious. The victim may hear a bone snap or see it pierce the skin. Often, however, not enough evidence exists to indicate whether a person has fractured a bone or simply sprained a muscle. People who suspect that they have broken a bone should have X-rays taken at a hospital.

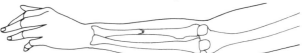

Closed fracture: *The broken bone does not pierce the skin.*

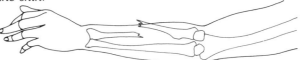

Open fracture: *The broken bone pierces the skin.*

Signs and symptoms: Fractures

1. Pain or tenderness in the injured area.
2. Loss of strength or inability to move an injured part.
3. Swelling or bruising.
4. Deformity or noticeable difference in the shape or length of the bone when it is compared to the same bone on the opposite limb.
5. A grating sensation in the injured area.

The skeletal system
Every bone in your body is part of the skeletal system. Your bones serve many functions: they protect delicate organs, store minerals, manufacture blood cells, provide a surface to which muscles and other structures attach, and act as levers that help you walk and move.

Dislocations

A dislocation occurs when the end of a bone separates from a joint such as the elbow, shoulder, finger, or thumb.

Signs and symptoms: Dislocations

1. Severe pain.
2. Inability to move joint.
3. Some deformity.
4. Swelling.

Procedure: Dislocations

1. Treat the injury as a fracture if you don't know whether the injury is a dislocation or a fracture.
2. Don't move the joint.
3. Don't try to put bones in a normal position.
4. Splint or immobilize the injured area in the position you find it.
5. If the injured area is the shoulder or elbow, have the victim put the affected arm close to his body, and immobilize the arm.
6. See a doctor.

Procedures: General bone injuries

1. Don't move the injured area.
2. Check the victim's airway and restore breathing and circulation if necessary.
3. Examine the victim for open wounds.
4. Stop any severe bleeding.
5. Treat the victim for shock if necessary.
6. If the victim is unconscious or shows symptoms of a serious head, neck, or back injury, don't move the victim. (See Head, Neck, and Spine Injuries, p. 27.)
7. Don't try to set or straighten the injured area.
8. If possible, use a splint to immobilize the injured part.
9. Elevate the injured area, and apply ice to help prevent swelling and bruising.
10. Don't give the victim anything by mouth.
11. Get medical attention.

Splinting

If the victim may have a fracture, use a splint to immobilize the injured area.
1. You can make a splint from rolled up newspapers or magazines, sticks, umbrellas, boards, pillows, or even the victim's other leg, if the injured part is a leg.
2. Make the splint long enough to extend past the joints above and below the possible broken bone.
3. Pad the splint with suitable soft material.
4. Tie the splint in place with bandages, neckties, belts, or strips of fabric.
5. Don't bind the splint tightly. Loosen the splint ties if the victim complains of tingling or numbness, if you cannot locate the victim's pulse, or if the victim's toes or fingers turn blue.
6. Do not delay medical treatment to make a complicated splint.

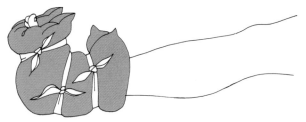

Splinting a broken foot: *Wrap and tie the injured foot in a pillow or cushioned material.*

Splinting broken bones

Broken lower arm

Do not cover the fingertips but keep them about 4 inches higher than the elbow.

Broken upper arm

Place the splint on the outside of the injured arm and either strap-support the forearm to the body or apply a sling.

Broken collarbone

Have the victim keep the arm on the injured side against his body as you apply a sling and bind the arm.

Broken jaw

Use nonadhesive cloth and slowly raise the victim's lower jaw.

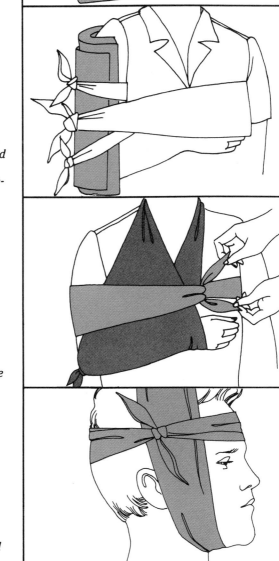

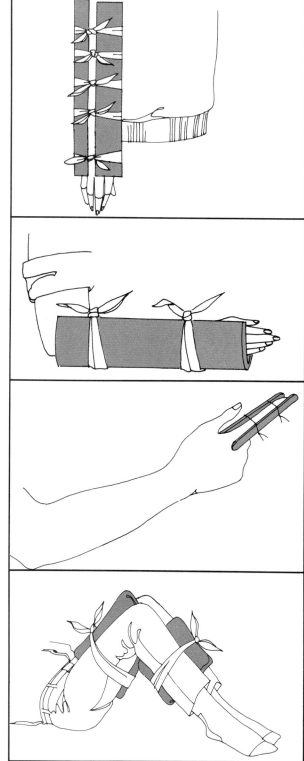

Broken elbow, with arm straight
Apply padded splints to both sides from the armpit to the fingers.

Broken elbow, with arm bent
Apply a sling and bind it firmly without cutting off circulation.

Broken finger
Keep the injured hand higher than the elbow.

Broken hip
Depending on which position is more comfortable, bend the victim's knees or keep them straight.

Broken knee
Place splint from buttocks to the area below the heel.

Broken lower leg
Place splint from above the knee to below the heel.

Broken upper leg
Tie legs together so uninjured leg acts as splint.

Burns

Preventing fires
- *Keep a fire extinguisher in the kitchen.*
- *Use appliances according to instructions.*
- *Don't overload electrical circuits.*
- *Keep matches out of a child's reach.*
- *Unplug appliances not in use.*
- *Fill kerosene heaters outdoors.*
- *Discard old oil cans and oily rags.*
- *Never smoke in bed.*
- *Never use spray cans near flames.*
- *Don't let newspapers or other papers pile up in the basement.*

How to deal with clothing on fire
- *If your clothes are on fire, lie down and roll on the ground. Flames will spread rapidly if you run about.*
- *If another person's clothes are on fire, smother the flames by wrapping the victim in a rug, blanket, or heavy piece of cloth. Don't use blankets or rugs made of synthetic material—they're highly flammable.*
- *Cool the victim's burns with water.*
- *Call an ambulance.*

A person may be burned by fire, dry or moist heat, steam, hot objects and liquids, chemicals, radiation, light, or electricity. Since the injured tissue resulting from a burn retains heat, tissue damage will continue until the burn victim cools the injured area. As a consequence, the victim should first work to cool the burn, thus preventing further tissue damage and easing the burn pain.

The severity and extent of a burn will help determine what treatment to give. A first- or second-degree burn involvoing a small portion of the victim's body (not including the face) represents a minor burn. If the hands, feet, or face are involved, the burn should be considered major; someone should call an ambulance. Burns to children and the elderly are always more serious. If a person has any doubt about a burn's severity, he should consider the burn to be major.

First-degree burns
If someone comes home from a sunny afternoon at the beach with red skin, which is not swollen or blistered, that person is suffering from a first-degree burn. Touching a hot object or scalding a small area of skin with steam also causes first-degree burns. First-degree burns don't cause deep tissue damage.

Signs and symptoms: First-degree burns
1. Redness.
2. Pain.

Procedure: First-degree burns
1. Apply cold, wet compresses to the burn, or soak the area in cold water for about ½ hour or until the pain subsides.
2. Cover the burn with a sterile dressing. For sunburn, apply Solarcaine or another over-the-counter preparation.

*Things to remember
when treating
second-degree burns*

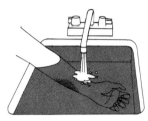

*1. Cool the burn with cold
running water or place the
burned area in a basin of
cold water.*

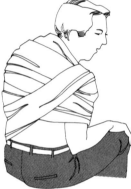

*2. Cover the burn with a
loose dressing.
3. If the victim's arms and
legs are burned, elevate
them.*

Second-degree burns

A person has a second-degree burn when the first layer of skin is burned through and the second layer is damaged. As a result, the victim suffers severe discomfort. Blisters and red, mottled skin accompany second-degree burns. Considerable swelling of the burned area will occur over several days, and fluids will ooze from the skin.

Signs and symptoms: Second-degree burns

1. Redness or blotchiness.
2. Swelling.
3. Severe pain.
4. Blistering and oozing.

Procedure: Second-degree burns

1. Cool the burned skin with cold running water, or place burned area in a basin of cold water. If neither is available, use cold, wet compresses.
2. Continue cooling until the pain diminishes.
3. Don't break blisters, or remove bits of skin.
4. Don't use antiseptic sprays or ointments on a severe burn.
5. Cover the burn area with a loose dressing.
6. Change the dressing if it becomes soaked with fluid oozing from the burn area.
7. If the victim's arms and legs are burned, elevate them.
8. Have the victim see a doctor immediately for second-degree burns of face, hands, or feet.

Third-degree burns

A third-degree burn may not hurt as much as a second-degree burn, because the damage to deep tissue destroys nerve endings. Fire and electric shock can cause third-degree burns. The burn may look white or charred or resemble a second-degree burn. All layers of skin will be damaged, and fat, muscle, and bone may also be damaged or exposed.

Signs and symptoms: Third-degree burns

1. White or charred skin.
2. Swelling.
3. Little or no pain.
4. The victim may be in shock.

Burn treatment:
Guidelines
- *Cool burned skin.*
- *Don't use cold water on large third-degree burns.*
- *Apply clean dressing.*
- *Keep the victim comfortable.*
- *Don't put ointments or home remedies on burns.*
- *Don't break blisters.*
- *Seek medical attention for all second- and third-degree burns.*

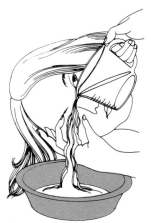

Pouring water
continuously
over an eye

Procedure: Third-degree burns

1. Call an ambulance immediately.
2. If the victim's legs or arms are burned, elevate them above the heart.
3. Use cold cloth compresses on burns of face, hands, and feet.
4. Treat the victim for symptoms of shock. (See Shock, p. 38.)
5. If the victim has face burns, have him sit up.
6. Cover the victim's burns with a clean dressing.
7. Don't apply antiseptic spray or ointment to the burned areas.
8. Don't put cold water on extensive burns—it may cause shock.

Chemical burns

Many household products contain strong chemicals, which should not be touched or inhaled. When accidents occur, these chemicals can cause serious burns. Chemical burns are major emergencies and require immediate action.

Procedure: Chemical burns

1. Flush the affected area with large quantities of water to rinse off the chemical and to prevent further damage. Use a shower or hose, if possible. Use running water for at least 5 to 10 mintues.
2. Remove the victim's clothing from the affected area as you continue to flush the skin with water.
3. Cover the burn with a clean dressing.
4. Get medical help quickly.

Procedure: Chemical burns of the eye

1. Get the victim to lie down. Hold his eyelids open with your index finger and thumb.
2. Pour water continuously over the eye, eyelids, and face.
3. Don't let the chemical run into the other eye.
4. Flush the eye for at least 15 minutes.
5. Don't rub the eye.
6. Cover the eye with a clean dressing.
7. Get immediate medical attention.

Childbirth

Supplies needed for childbirth
- *Clean cotton sheets.*
- *Blankets.*
- *Plastic bag for the placenta, or afterbirth.*
- *Clean cloth or sanitary napkins.*
- *Clean, strong string to tie the umbilical cord, for example, a shoelace.*
- *Scissors.*
- *Soap and water.*

Childbirth is a natural process. The labor accompanying childbirth usually spans enough time to allow the woman sufficient opportunity to reach the hospital. Labor may start, however, unexpectedly or progress rapidly, and the woman may give birth before reaching the hospital. In such circumstances, the woman would greatly benefit from knowledgeable assistance.

Signs and symptoms: Impending childbirth

1. Labor pains occur approximately two minutes apart and the woman feels the urge to push downward in an effort to expel the baby. (Labor pains, or contractions, result from the tightening and relaxing of the uterus muscles.)
2. The bag of water has broken. (Until childbirth, an amniotic sac filled with fluid protects the fetus. In the early stage of labor, the sac usually breaks, expelling the amniotic fluid, allowing fetus to pass through birth canal.)
3. The woman cries out constantly or warns that the baby is coming.
4. The baby's head may be visible at the vaginal opening at the time of a contraction.

Procedure: Childbirth

1. Call a doctor or take the woman to the hospital as quickly as possible.
2. Wash your hands with soap and water.
3. If help is unlikely to arrive and you can't get to a hospital, prepare for the delivery in a quiet place. Cover the bed or other delivery surface with a clean blanket or towel. If possible, place a plastic sheet underneath the blanket. Have the pregnant woman remove all her clothes below the waist and have her lie down with her knees bent, feet flat on the surface on which she is resting, her thighs separated widely. (If you're in a car, have the pregnant woman lie down on the back seat with one leg on the floor and the other on the back seat.)

Support the baby as he emerges.

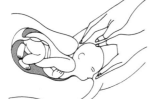

Support the head

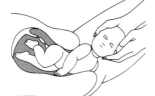

Aid in the delivery of the upper shoulder

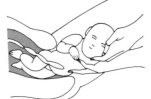

Support the trunk

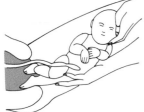

Support the legs

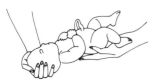

Position for drainage

4. Inspect the vaginal opening to see if the baby's head is visible at the time of a contraction. If the head is visible, birth will probably occur shortly.

5. Ask the mother not to push or bear down on her stomach, but pant instead. Don't place your fingers or hands in the woman's vagina.

6. To prevent the baby's head from coming out too quickly, place gentle pressure on the head as it emerges.

7. If the bag of water isn't broken and covers the baby's face, quickly puncture the bag to allow the fluid to escape. Use your fingers to tear the bag if you don't have a blunt object. Then pull the membranes away from the baby's face.

8. As the baby's head emerges, support it with both hands but don't try to slow down or speed up the delivery by pushing or pulling the baby. Note the umbilical cord's placement. If the umbilical cord is wrapped around the baby's neck, gently work the cord over the baby's head. In rare cases, you may have to cut the umbilical cord if it is too tight to slip over the baby's head. If you must cut the cord to prevent the baby from choking, tie the cord in two places with string, and cut between the ties.

9. As the baby emerges, continue to support his head. The baby's shoulders will emerge with the next contraction, so tell the mother to breathe quickly four times and then to push hard. When the shoulders appear, gently guide the baby's head downward to facilitate the delivery of the upper shoulder. With the next contraction, guide the baby's head upward for the lower shoulder's delivery. Do not force the baby in either direction.

10. Tell the mother to push hard once more to deliver the rest of the baby. Remember, a newborn baby is very slippery, so support it firmly but gently with one hand cupping his head and the other grasping his buttocks or feet as they emerge.

11. Support the baby firmly with his head down to drain the mucus from his mouth and nose. Wipe the baby's nose and mouth with a clean cloth or gauze.

Use string to tie off umbilical cord after the baby is born.

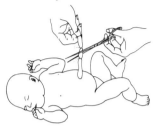

Special considerations: The baby

1. If the baby doesn't start breathing on his own, assist by gently rubbing the baby's back or the soles of his feet until he starts to cry.

2. If the baby doesn't respond, stroke his throat from neck to chin, then sweep your finger into the baby's mouth to clear any mucus. If the baby still isn't breathing, give mouth-to-nose resuscitation. Use gentle puffs, 1 every 5 seconds. (See Artificial Respiration, pp. 20-21.)

3. Keep the baby warm by quickly wiping him dry, placing him stomach-down on his mother's abdomen, and covering him entirely, including his head, leaving only his face exposed.

4. Tie the umbilical cord in two places (see illustration) and cover it to keep it clean. Don't cut the cord.

Special considerations: The mother

1. Contractions will resume soon after the baby's birth. These contractions are the preparation for the expulsion of the placenta, commonly called the afterbirth.

WARNING: Don't try to hasten this natural process by pulling the umbilical cord or by pressing on the mother's abdomen. Since the placenta may be delivered up to 30 minutes after the baby's delivery, get the mother to a hospital as soon as possible. You do not have to wait for the placenta.

2. If you see signs of placenta delivery (umbilical cord lengthening or blood gushing from the vagina), tell the mother to push hard as you apply downward pressure on her lower abdomen.

3. Once the placenta emerges, you can control bleeding by massaging the mother's uterus. To do so, place your hand on her lower abdomen and massage it gently but firmly. You'll feel the uterus firm up when you do this. Repeat the massage every 5 minutes for 1 hour or until assistance arrives.

4. Save the placenta in a plastic bag or towel and take it to the hospital with the mother and baby.

5. Cleanse the vaginal opening with a moist towel and place a clean cloth or sanitary napkin over the vaginal opening.

WARNING: Don't try to deliver a baby whose foot, arm, shoulder, or buttocks appear first. Get the mother to the hospital immediately.

Place the baby on the mother's chest or abdomen to help keep the baby warm and to keep the mother and baby close.

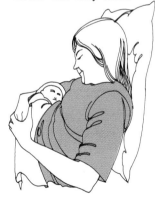

Cold Exposure

A person with frostbitten hands or feet must regularly exercise the hurt parts to improve circulation.

For the feet:

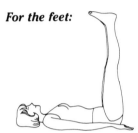

1. Raise the legs overhead for 2 minutes.

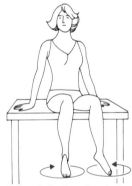

2. Swirl the legs in circles for 2 minutes.

For the hands:

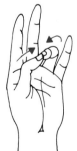

1. Touch the tip of the thumb with each finger.

Your toes, fingers, nose, and ears are the body parts most often affected by frostbite. Exposure to very low temperature or high winds on cold days causes the fluid in skin and tissue cells to form ice crystals.

Signs and symptoms: Frostbite

1. Red skin in early stages turning white or grayish-yellow.
2. A feeling of coldness and numbness in affected areas.
3. Blisters form 12 to 24 hours after exposure.
4. Possible sharp pain in early stages; skin may later feel hard.

Procedure: Frostbite

1. Call an ambulance.
2. Cover the affected area. The victim can hold his hands next to his body for extra warmth.
3. Get the victim to a warm place.
4. Immerse the affected area in warm water (about 100° F.). If warm water is not available, gently wrap the area in a blanket. (Rewarming will be very painful.)
5. Don't rub the frostbitten area. Don't use hot water bottles, stoves, or radiators to warm the victim.
6. Don't break blisters.
7. When the victim's skin returns to a normal color, stop the warming process.

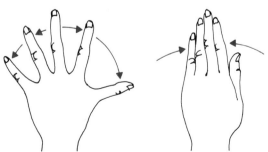

2. Spread the fingers; then squeeze them together.

How to prevent hypothermia

• *In cold, wet weather, or cool, windy weather, wear warm clothing and water repellent outer garments and boots. Staying dry is important.*
• *Don't drink alcoholic beverages before you go out in the cold. Alcohol increases the loss of body heat.*
• *Avoid getting overheated when you are outdoors. The moisture of the perspiration takes away body heat.*
• *If you get chilled, go indoors for at least two hours.*
• *During a long, very cold spell, eat a diet high in fats and carbohydrates.*
• *If you work or play outdoors in winter, dress adequately. Keep your head, hands, ears, and feet well-covered. Wear double layers on your hands and feet.*
• *If you're 65 years or older, keep the indoor temperature at 65° F. or more, especially when you're inactive.*

8. Put sterile gauze between frostbitten fingers and toes.
9. Give the victim warm liquids but no alcoholic beverages. Don't apply additional heat or allow the victim to sit near a radiator, stove, or fire.
10. Keep the frostbitten areas elevated.
11. Get medical assistance.

Hypothermia

Long exposure to a cold temperature or to a cool, windy environment may affect the entire body. The victim's temperature will fall below normal.

Signs and symptoms: Hypothermia

1. Shivering.
2. Numbness.
3. Reduced body temperature.
4. Muscle weakness or poor coordination.
5. Drowsiness or sluggishness.
6. Possible slurred speech.

Procedure: Hypothermia

1. Call an ambulance.
2. Move the victim to a warm area as soon as possible.
3. Give artificial respiration if necessary. (See Artificial Respiration, pp. 20-21.)
4. Remove wet or frozen clothes. Wrap the victim in blankets.
5. If the victim is conscious, give him warm liquids but no alcoholic beverages.
6. Follow the procedure for frostbite if the victim also has areas of frostbite.

Dental Emergencies

Wrap the victim's knocked-out tooth in a wet cloth. If possible, carry the tooth in a cup of cold milk, which will help preserve the tooth more effectively than water. A dentist may be able to replant the tooth if the root has not been too severely damaged.

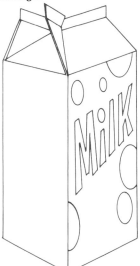

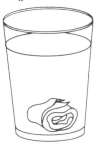

A young boy and his friends are playing hockey. In front of the goal, they scramble for the puck. A stick comes up too high and hits the boy in the mouth. One of his upper front teeth falls out, and several other teeth are chipped. The boy's friends can do several things to help him.

Procedure: Knocked-out tooth

1. Check the victim's mouth for bleeding. Remove any pieces of broken tooth.
2. If the gum is bleeding, place a gauze pad, a clean handkerchief, or a tissue over the wound. Have the victim hold the pad tightly in place.
3. Wrap the knocked-out tooth in a wet cloth.
4. Take the victim and the tooth to the dentist as quickly as possible.

Toothache

Sunday morning Carol woke up with a terrible throbbing in her mouth. How can she take care of the toothache until she can get to the dentist?

Causes of toothaches

A toothache may be caused by a cavity or an infection. The infection could be located between the tooth and the gum, at the root of the tooth, in the tooth's pulp, or in the sinuses.

Procedure: Toothache

1. Let the victim take aspirin or aspirin substitute to relieve the pain.
2. Hold an ice pack to the victim's jaw to relieve the pain.
3. Avoid extremely hot or cold liquids.
4. Call a dentist or visit the emergency room of your hospital. Most emergency room doctors can examine mouths.

Drowning

Ways to prevent drowning

- *Wherever you swim, obey all rules and warning notices.*
- *Teach children to swim as early as possible.*
- *Don't let young children play in boats without an adult present.*
- *Don't let young children swim or bathe unless they are supervised.*
- *Don't swim alone.*
- *Don't dive into water if you don't know how deep it is or if you can't see the bottom.*

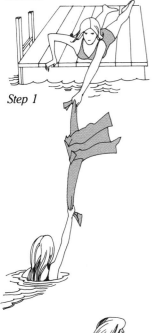

Step 1

Step 2

No one should swim out to rescue a drowning person unless he is trained in lifesaving. A drowning person in deep water may grab his rescuer, endangering both their lives. Because most drownings occur near shore, a rescuer can usually use non-swimming methods.

Procedure: Water rescue

1. If the victim is near shore, reach out to him with a towel, oar, pole, or rope.
2. If the victim is farther away from shore, wade out to him. Take an oar, board, or other object that the victim can grasp.
3. Whenever possible, have a partner help you with an attempted rescue. If the victim is in deeper water, reach him by rowboat, if possible. Instruct the victim to hold onto the stern of the boat while you row to shore. If the victim can't hold onto the boat, have your partner assist you in getting the victim into the boat. Check the victim for injuries while your partner rows ashore.
4. Clear the victim's airway, and begin artificial respiration immediately. (See Artificial Respiration, pp. 20-21.)
5. Check the victim's carotid pulse. If you can't feel a pulse, ask a professionally trained person to begin cardiac compression.
6. Keep the victim warm and check for signs of shock. (See Shock, pp. 38-45.)
7. Call an ambulance.

Ice rescue

A rescuer should warn a person who has fallen through the ice not to struggle or try to climb out. Moving about may break the ice a second time. Speed is important in an ice rescue but so is the safety of both victim and rescuer.

Procedure: Ice rescue

1. Use a light ladder to reach the victim. Lie on the ladder while another person pushes it and you over the ice toward the victim. Have the victim hold onto the ladder while you or another person pulls it back to shore.

2. If a ladder is not available, use a pole, stick, board, rope, or buoy to reach the victim. If only people are available, make a human chain. Spread your weight out over as large an area as possible.

3. Slide the victim to shore on his stomach.

4. Get the victim to a warm area. Give artificial respiration if necessary.

5. Check for signs of shock. Call a doctor.

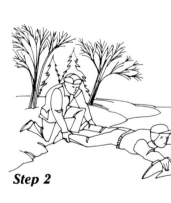

Step 1

Step 2

Drug Overdose

A drug is any substance other than food that affects the mind or body when taken into the body. Any drug, even a prescription medication, can be dangerous when not used according to instructions.

Joe suspected that his sister Elizabeth had overdosed on drugs. He immediately called an ambulance, then tried to identify the substance. Joe checked his sister's eyes for frequent blinking, rapid eye movements, and pinpoint or dilated pupils. He then checked her forearms for needle marks. He asked her which drugs she had taken. While waiting for the ambulance, Joe also looked for hypodermic needles, eye droppers, cigarette papers, vials, capsules, or other drug apparatus. He knew that anything he found would help the doctor or emergency personnel in deciding the correct treatment for his sister.

Procedure: Drug overdose

If you suspect that someone you know has overdosed on drugs, you should follow these general rules.

1. Keep the airway open.
2. Give artificial respiration if necessary. (See Artificial Respiration, pp. 20-21.)
3. Maintain the victim's body temperature.
4. Try to determine what drugs were taken.
5. Make sure that the victim can't hurt himself or others.
6. You may suspect that the victim has taken only alcohol. If so, check breathing, pulse, and color. If these signs are normal, let the victim sleep. Cold, clammy skin, rapid pulse, and abnormal breathing are signs of shock. If these signs appear, treat the victim and get medical help. (See Shock, pp. 38-45.)
7. Keep the victim from hurting himself or others and keep him calm, if possible.
8. Get medical help.

Ear Injuries

Objects in the ear

Children sometimes put common objects such as beans, beads, paper, and cotton into their ears. Insects sometimes find their way into the ears of children and adults alike.

Procedure:
Objects in the ear

1. The buzzing of an insect trapped in the ear may panic the victim. You can kill the insect by putting a few drops of oil (baby, mineral, or cooking) into the ear. Only use oil for an insect. Have a doctor remove the insect.

2. Have a doctor remove any object. Don't let the victim hit his head to dislodge the object.

3. If paper or cotton is clearly visible at the opening of the victim's ear canal, remove it carefully with your fingers, if possible.

4. Don't put anything into the canal. The doctor will make sure no material remains inside the ear.

Blood or other fluids coming from inside the ear may indicate a cut in the ear canal or a ruptured eardrum. A ruptured eardrum can result from an extremely loud sound, a blow to the head, a change in pressure (as in diving), an ear infection, or an object pushed into your ear. When bleeding from the ear occurs, you may not be able to tell if the injury is a cut or a ruptured eardrum. Follow the general procedure for ear injuries.

Signs and symptoms: Ear injuries

1. Bleeding.
2. Pain.
3. Hearing loss.

Procedure: Ear injuries

1. If the victim has a head injury, treat that injury first. (See Head, Neck, and Spine Injuries, pp. 27-30.)
2. Don't put anything into the ear.
3. Don't try to stop the bleeding. Cover the outer ear with a bandage or a clean cloth. Tape the bandage loosely in place.
4. Have the victim lie down with the injured ear facing down to allow the blood to drain.
5. Get medical help.

Earache

An earache is usually caused by an infection. For example, bacteria from a common cold can travel from the nose and throat through the Eustachian tube and infect the middle ear. Swimming in contaminated water is another major cause of ear infection.

Signs and symptoms: Earache

1. Pain.
2. Fever.
3. Possible discharge from the ear.

Procedure: Earache

1. Don't use drops without the advice of a doctor. Have a doctor examine the victim's ear.
2. Don't use a cotton swab or any other object to clean out the victim's ear.
3. Let the victim take aspirin or aspirin substitute to relieve the pain.
4. Call a doctor.

Eye Injuries

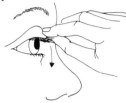

*1. Have the person look
down. Grasp the lashes of
the upper lid and pull up.*

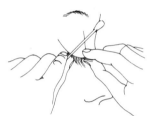

*2. Place a cotton swab stick
or similar object across the
lid, pull the lashes out and
up over the stick.*

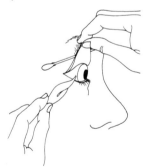

*3. When you see the speck,
gently remove it with the
corner of a wet cloth or tissue.
4. If necessary, check under
the lower lid by pulling it
down.*

A blow near the eye can break small blood vessels beneath the skin. The skin swells and becomes discolored. The result is a "black eye".

Procedure: Blunt injuries

1. An ice pack or cold compress will reduce pain and swelling of the victim's eye.
2. Take the victim to a doctor.

Foreign objects in the eye

You can safely remove an eyelash, cinder, or other small speck that gets into the eye. Larger particles that can scratch the eye's surface, or objects that are imbedded in the eye, should get immediate medical attention.

Signs and symptoms: Foreign objects in the eye

1. Pain and redness.
2. Burning and tearing.

Procedure: Foreign objects in the eye

1. Do not let the victim rub his eyes.
2. Wash your hands before examining the victim's eyes.
3. Cover both eyes with a sterile compress. Tie the compress in place lightly.
4. Keep the victim on his back, if possible.
5. Get the victim to a doctor.

Procedure: Small particles in the eye

1. Pull the upper lid down over the lower lid. In a moment, the victim's eyes should begin to water. The tears may wash out the particle.
2. If the particle remains, fill a medicine dropper with warm water and gently flush the eye.
3. Flushing with water may not remove the particle. Pull down the lower lid. If the particle is visible, remove it with the corner of a wet cloth or tissue.
4. If the particle remains, cover the eye with a clean, dry cloth and get the victim to a doctor.
5. Even if the injury seems minor, take the victim to a doctor because there may be bleeding or injury that you cannot see inside the eye.

Fainting

Anyone who feels faint should sit with the head lowered to knee level.

Y ou may faint or lose consciousness if the supply of blood to your brain is reduced for a short time. Physical or emotional shock, pain, hunger, and fear can make you faint. Fainting can be prevented by lying down or sitting down and putting your head lower than knee level.

Signs and symptoms: Fainting

1. Sweating.
2. Clammy skin.
3. Paleness.
4. Dizziness.
5. Nausea.

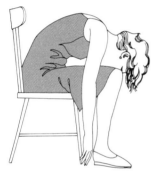

Procedure: Fainting

1. Have the victim lie on his back. Elevate the victim's feet about 12 inches.
2. Loosen tight clothing.
3. If the victim vomits, turn his head to the side to keep his air passage clear.
4. Hold a cool, wet cloth to the victim's face. Don't pour water over the victim's face.
5. Don't give the victim any liquids until he has recovered.
6. Call an ambulance if the victim does not recover in a few minutes.
7. After the victim regains consciousness, keep him lying down for about 10 minutes. Advise the victim to get up slowly.

Caution: Anyone who faints should be examined by a doctor. The fainting may be a symptom of an undiagnosed disorder.

Fever

Using a thermometer

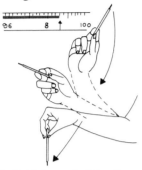

1. Hold the end of the thermometer opposite the bulb. Shake the thermometer until the silver (or red) line moves below 98.6° F.

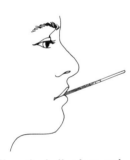

2. Place the bulb of an oral thermometer under the victim's tongue. Make sure that the victim keeps his mouth closed for at least 3 to 4 minutes. If the victim has had a hot bath, has smoked, or has had hot or cold food or liquids, wait at least a half hour before taking his temperature.

Fever is usually a sign that the body is fighting an infection. During an illness or infection, a fever is normal and may help the body overcome the disorder; however, a very high fever, a fever that lasts several days, or one accompanied by nausea, chills, pain, or rash can be harmful.

Average normal temperature is 98.6° F., although a person's temperature may be slightly higher or lower. Also, a person's temperature usually rises slightly in the evening.

Signs and symptoms: Fever
1. Temperature higher than normal.
2. Possible weakness, heavy sweating, and headache.

Procedure: Adults
1. Take the victim's temperature. If the victim's temperature is 101° F. or higher, continue taking the temperature every half hour. Keep a record of the victim's temperature.
2. Remove extra bed covers or excess clothes. The victim should be comfortable but not chilly.
3. Let the victim take aspirin or aspirin substitute to bring the fever down.
4. A sponge bath with warm water will help bring the fever down.
5. If the fever continues or rises rapidly, call a doctor.

Procedure: Children
1. Take the child's temperature every half hour.
2. Call a doctor when a child's temperature rises over 101° F. High fever in infants and young children may lead to convulsions.
3. Check with a doctor before giving the child any medication for fever.
4. Have the child rest and drink liquids.
5. Give the child a sponge bath with warm water. Don't use alcohol.

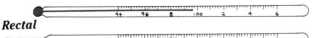

Rectal

Oral

3. A rectal temperature reading will be about 1° higher than an oral temperature. Normal rectal temperature is 99.6° F.

Fits (Convulsions)

All movements, senses, and thinking are controlled by the brain. Usually, the areas of the brain work together smoothly. If, however, an electrical disturbance occurs within a person's brain and some cells become more active than normal, the person may become unconscious. The period of unconsciousness may be accompanied by a convulsion or seizure. During a seizure, a rigidity of the persons' muscles is followed by violent muscular movement, drooling or foaming at the mouth, and discoloration of the face. The person can sustain an injury during a convulsion from hitting hard objects as he falls or thrashes about.

Convulsions may be caused by a head injury, brain disease, brain tumor, high fever, an acute infection, eclampsia (a condition that can develop in late stages of pregnancy), or a chronic disease known as epilepsy.

Signs and symptoms: Convulsions
1. The victim loses consciousness.
2. The victim's eyes may roll, he may drool, his muscles may stiffen and twitch, and he may have facial discoloration as a result of a temporary loss of breathing.

Procedure: Convulsions
1. Try to catch the victim as he is falling, and lay him down.
2. Move any sharp objects, furniture, or other items on which the victim might injure himself while thrashing about.
3. Check the victim's breathing. Maintain an open airway and give artificial respiration, if necessary. (If the attack is prolonged, breathing may stop.)
4. Don't put anything in the victim's mouth.
5. Don't try to stop the convulsion.
6. Loosen any tight clothing.
7. Don't throw liquids into the victim's mouth or on his face.
8. When the convulsion stops, keep the victim lying down, but turn him on his side to prevent choking.
9. Call an ambulance.
10. Check the victim for injuries.

Convulsions in children
When a baby or young child has a convulsion because of a high fever:
• *Prevent injury.*
• *Loosen tight clothing.*
• *Don't place the child in a tub of water to reduce fever.*
• *Reduce fever by sponging with lukewarm water.*
• *Call a doctor.*

Headaches

More people seek treatment for headaches than for any other medical problem. A headache may come from tension, an allergy, illness, or eye problems—or it may be a disorder itself, like a migraine headache.

J oanna Wallace, age 32, knew exactly when her problem began. She had just received some good news about a job promotion. She ran to her office to make a phone call and suddenly became dreadfully ill. A sharp pain began in her forehead and quickly radiated to the back of her head. Then she vomited violently. Joanna had never experienced such sharp head pain and sudden nausea before, nor did she suffer from chronic headaches. On the following day the headache pain had settled behind her right eye as well. How should Joanna's headache be treated?

Nearly everyone feels a headache throb at one time or another. In fact, more people seek treatment for headaches than for any other medical problem. In rare cases, the headache is a warning symptom of some disease. In most cases, however, the headache results from muscle tension, an allergy, minor illness, or eye disorders. In some instances, the headache is part of a disorder (or a syndrome) that doctors describe as migraine headaches.

Tension headaches

In most cases, stress or a combination of psychological factors produces a tension headache. Anxiety, depression, and anger can cause painful, sustained muscle contraction in the head—the source of many headaches.

The tension headache victim may have pain in any part of the head: the temples, forehead, back, or top of the head. A sense of weight, a pulling, a bandlike or caplike pressure are but a few of the terms people use to describe tension headaches.

Procedure: Tension headaches

1. Let the victim take aspirin or aspirin substitute for relief of pain.
2. Massage the victim's neck muscles, temples, and scalp.
3. Have the victim rest in a quiet place.
4. Apply a cold compress to the victim's head.

The procedures for tension headaches will also help headaches that are associated with fever and flu. If the victim is a chronic sufferer of tension headaches, he may benefit from biofeedback training at a headache clinic.

The pain process

No matter what type of headache you have, the first step in the pain process is the stimulation of an electrical impulse in sensitive nerve endings. The stimulation is both chemical and electrical. The pain alters the electrical charge of molecules at the sensitive end of a nerve fiber. The change in the electrical charge creates an electrical impulse that travels along the nerve fiber. At the other end of the nerve fiber, chemicals stimulate a pain signal in a nearby nerve. The process continues from nerve to nerve, to the spinal column, and then to the brain where the pain is interpreted.

At any step in the process, a painkiller can block or cancel the pain message.

Signs and symptoms: Migraine headaches

The victim of a migraine headache experiences warning signs. Most frequently the warnings are visual: flashing lights, patterns, areas of darkness, or zigzag lines. A feeling of weakness in one or more limbs, slight confusion, dizziness, drowsiness, and uncertainty of gait are other warnings.

Migraine headaches, which tend to occur in the morning, may begin up to 30 minutes after the first warning signs. The headache usually hits one side of the head; one-sidedness is characteristic of the migraine headache.

Once the headache begins, the victim commonly loses his appetite and feels nauseated. Vomiting may also occur. The victim's eyes may redden and swell, and his nasal passages may feel stuffy. He may also have an aversion to light.

Procedure: Migraine headaches

1. During the migraine attack, have the victim lie down in a darkened room.
2. Elevate the victim's head slightly.
3. When the attack has subsided, have the victim rest for a while.
4. Have the victim keep a record of the migraine attacks to see if a pattern emerges.
5. Have the victim see a doctor so that he can evaluate the migraine pattern and prescribe treatment to help control the attacks.
6. Have the victim follow the doctor's recommendations faithfully.

Caution: Regardless of prior headache experiences, have the victim seek medical attention immediately if he experiences any of the following:

- **A headache following a blow to the head.**
- **A sudden headache with no apparent cause.**
- **Chronic headaches that interfere with the victim's normal pattern of living.**
- **A headache associated with a particular part of the head, such as an eye or ear.**
- **Recurrent headaches, especially in a child.**

Heat Exposure

Exposure to excessive heat can affect the body in a variety of ways that will result in an emergency. Heat cramps, heat exhaustion, and heat stroke are conditions resulting from response to heat. Heat-related illness is always more serious if the victim is a child, is an older person, has a chronic illness, or is injured. The severity of a heat reaction depends on the victim's body temperature, the amount of circulating air around the victim, the humidity of the environment, and the type and amount of clothing worn by the victim.

Heat exhaustion

Heat exhaustion is a response to heat resulting from loss of body fluids and salt through sweating or inadequate intake of fluids.

When people lose a large amount of salt and body fluids, they may suffer heat exhaustion.

Signs and symptoms: Heat exhaustion
1. Normal or slightly elevated temperature.
2. Pale, clammy skin.
3. Heavy sweating.
4. Weakness, dizziness, fainting, or nausea.

Procedure: Heat exhaustion
1. Move the victim to a cool area. Have the victim lie down and elevate his feet.
2. Loosen the victim's clothing.
3. Have the victim drink half a glass of water every 15 minutes for 1 hour, unless the victim vomits. Don't give liquids to unconscious victims.
4. Apply cool, wet compresses and fan the victim.
5. If the symptoms get worse or last more than 1 hour, call a doctor.

Caution: Increasing your intake of salt cannot protect you from heat exhaustion or heatstroke. Drinking adequate fluids and exercising sensibly can. Extra salt can elevate your blood pressure.

Heatstroke

Heatstroke is a response to heat that results when the body's heat-regulating mechanism fails. The victim's body temperature rises dangerously. Because the body's heat control fails, the victim may feel hot and dry, rather than wet from sweating.

Symptoms: Heatstroke

1. Extremely high body temperature.
2. Hot, red skin; possibly with no sweating.
3. Strong, rapid pulse.
4. Alterations in consciousness ranging from confusion to unconsciousness.

Procedure: Heatstroke

1. Call an ambulance immediately.
2. Put the undressed victim in a tub of cold water, sponge or wrap him in cool wet towels or sheets.
3. Check the victim's temperature often. Continue the cooling procedure until the victim's temperature falls below 102° F.
4. Use fans to cool the victim.
5. Don't give the victim alcoholic beverages or stimulants such as coffee or tea.

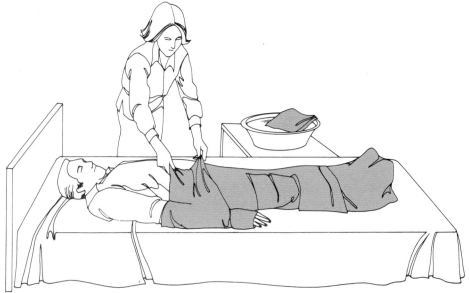

Placing wet sheets on a heatstroke victim.

Mouth Injuries

Three-year old Dennis received a cut on his mouth and on his tongue when he slipped and fell on the newly waxed floor. Mouth injuries that cause severe bleeding may also result in breathing difficulty if the blood goes down the throat.

Symptoms: Mouth injuries
1. Lips may be swollen and other visible signs may appear, such as an open wound on the lips, tongue, or the inside of the cheek.
2. Bleeding from the lips, tongue, gums, or the roof of the mouth may occur.
3. A tooth may be knocked out.

Procedure: Mouth injuries
1. If the victim has difficulty breathing, clear the airway and give artificial respiration, if necessary. (See Artificial Respiration, pp. 20-21.)
2. To control severe bleeding in the mouth, have the victim sit up and lean forward so that the blood can drain from his mouth. Then, use a sterile or clean cloth to apply direct pressure on the source of the bleeding.
3. See a doctor if you can't control bleeding or if the wound is large or deep.

Blood may be a problem
Mouth injuries often produce heavy bleeding, which may make the wound look more serious than it is. But the bleeding can be a problem.

Swallowed blood can lead to nausea and vomiting. Inhaled blood can lead to coughing, choking, and serious consequences like pneumonia.

To avoid these problems, have the bleeding victim lean forward so that the blood drains out of the mouth. Then, use a sterile or clean cloth to apply direct pressure on the source of the bleeding.

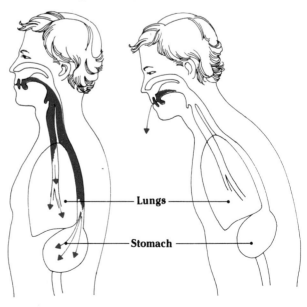

Lungs

Stomach

Muscle Cramps

Mrs. Rowen often wakes up during the night with a cramp in the ball of her foot. The toes on her aching foot curl up as the muscle tightens. What could be the cause of her muscle cramps?

A muscle cramp is a painful, sustained muscle contraction. Fatigue, poor circulation, an injury to the muscle, too much exercise, or cold are among the causes of muscle cramps.

Signs and symptoms: Muscle cramps
1. Sudden pain.
2. Tightness in the muscle.

Procedure: Muscle cramps
1. Help the victim stretch the affected muscle. If the victim's calf muscle is cramped, have him straighten his knee and pull the foot upward. If the cramp is in the leg or foot, help the victim walk around to relieve the spasm.

How to relieve a cramp in the calf
1. Straighten the victim's leg.
2. Push the victim's foot back. (If you have the cramp, pull the foot back yourself.)

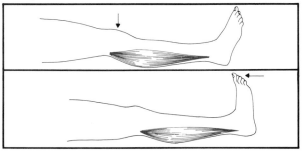

2. Massage the muscle using pressure rather than lightly rubbing.
3. Apply a warm compress.
Caution: A person who gets cramps frequently should see a doctor.

Muscle sprains
Gene turned his ankle when he stepped off the curb. His foot seemed to bend inward at the ankle as he fell, and the pain was intense. Gene probably sprained his ankle.

A sprain is an injury to a ligament or a joint. Some of the ligament fibers get torn. Stretching a joint beyond its normal range of motion can cause a sprain.

Not everyone can tell the difference between a sprain and a fracture. Small bones around the joints

Heat cramps
Heat cramps are painful muscle spasms in the most strenuously used muscles, such as thighs and shoulders. Sodium (salt) loss from perspiring or inadequate salt intake causes the cramps. Heat cramps usually occur during very hot weather. (See Heat Exposure, pp. 79-80.)

Symptoms: Heat cramps
1. Painful cramps.
2. Possible nausea, cool and pallid skin.

Procedure: Heat cramps
1. Let the victim sip water or a balanced electrolyte drink, such as Gatorade.
2. Have the victim lie down in a cool place.
3. Massage the muscle gently or try to relieve pain by placing your hands firmly on the muscle and exerting pressure.
Caution: Do not increase your salt intake without consulting a doctor.

can crack in minor accidents, and the only way to confirm or rule out a fracture is with an X-ray.

Signs and symptoms: Muscle sprains
1. Intense pain upon moving the joint.
2. Swelling and bruising of surrounding tissue.
3. Inability to move the joint.
4. Tenderness in the injured area.

Procedure: Muscle sprains
1. Immobilize the joint with a splint until the victim sees a doctor to rule out or confirm a fracture. (See Fractures, pp. 55-59, to find out how to splint injured joints.)
2. Loosen the splint if swelling makes it tight.
3. Apply an ice pack for about 48 hours. Leave the ice pack on for 15 to 20 minutes at a time. Then, remove it for 15 to 20 minues before reapplying.
4. After the swelling is under control, use warm compresses.
5. Have the victim elevate the injured joint above the level of the heart.

Muscle strain
Anyone who lifts heavy objects incorrectly or exerts himself doing new exercises knows what muscle strain feels like. A strain is a tearing or overstretching of muscle fibers. (See also Back Strain, p. 49.)

Signs and symptoms: Muscle strain
1. Sudden severe pain at the time of the injury.
2. Possible swelling around the strained muscle.
3. Chronic strain produces gradual onset of stiffness, soreness, and tenderness.

Procedure: Muscle strain
1. Have the victim rest the affected muscles.
2. If the strain is in a limb, have the victim elevate it above the heart.
3. Gently massage the affected area.
4. For acute strain, apply ice pack for the first 48 hours to control swelling. Leave the ice pack on for 15 to 20 minutes at a time. Then, remove it for 15 to 20 minutes before reapplying.
5. Apply warm compresses or use a heating pad when swelling is under control. Allow only minimal movement of the affected area.
6. Have the victim see a doctor for severe strain.

Nosebleed

Allergies, colds, overuse of nosedrops, blowing the nose too hard, or banging one's nose can cause severe nosebleeds. Nosebleeds can be a serious symptom when blood pressure is dangerously high, when the nosebleed is the result of a blow to the head, or when the bleeding is severe.

Procedure: Nosebleed

1. If bleeding is severe, call an ambulance while you start first aid.

2. Unless you suspect a serious head or neck injury, have the victim sit up and lean forward so that blood does not drip down his throat.

3. Have the victim use his thumb and forefinger to pinch his nostrils for about 10 minutes.

4. If the victim is using his hand for the direct pressure, you can apply cold compresses to the nose at the same time.

5. Have the victim breathe through his mouth during the direct pressure and for about 1 hour after the bleeding stops.

6. If bleeding continues after 10 or 15 minutes of direct pressure, gently pack the nostrils with clean cloth or with sterile gauze, and have the victim pinch his nostrils for another 5 minutes. Be sure to have a free end of the packing so that you can easily remove it. (Do not pack nostrils if you suspect a nasal fracture.)

7. Get medical help if the bleeding continues or if bleeding starts again.

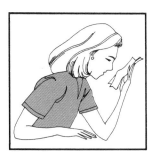

Step 2

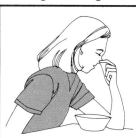

Step 3

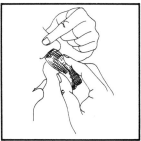

Step 6

Nose Injuries

Benefits of nasal breathing

Breathing through the nose moisturizes and warms the air, and removes dust particles before the air reaches the lungs. If a person can't breathe through the nose, these benefits are lost. Dry, cold, unfiltered air will reach the lungs through the mouth, leading to respiratory problems.

Foreign objects in the nose can damage the lining of the passages, interfering with breathing. Broken bones or displaced cartilage will produce swelling, tenderness, and probably discoloration. Untreated, these injuries can make normal breathing impossible.

Nose injury: Foreign object in the nose

Young children tend to put objects such as beads and peas in their nostrils. Even an adult may accidentally get a foreign object in his nose. No one should try to remove a foreign object lodged in a nostril unless the object is sticking out.

Procedure: Foreign object in the nose

1. Calm the victim.
2. Have the victim breathe through his mouth to avoid inhaling the object.
3. If the victim can blow his nose, have him try to expel the object.
4. Have the victim see a doctor if the object remains lodged in the nose.

Nose injury: Broken nose

Carrie stepped on a rake lying in her garden, and the rake handle hit her in the face. Her nose started to bleed immediately, but it did not begin to swell for several hours. Carrie probably broke her nose.

Symptoms: Broken nose

1. Possible distortion of the nose.
2. Swelling and bruising.
3. Tenderness.
4. Possible bleeding.

Procedure: Broken nose

1. Treat bleeding (See Nosebleed, p. 84.)
2. Don't pack the victim's nose.
3. Have the victim see a doctor immediately.

Splinter

*Splinters are not only pain-
ful; if they are not removed
quickly, or if the wound is
not properly cleaned, they
can cause serious infection.*

*If the splinter is deeply
embedded, don't 'dig' for it;
cleanse the area, apply a
clean dressing pad and
seek medical help.*

Kyra Nathan got some splinters in her left hand as she was carrying some firewood from the garage. The first thing she did was wash her hands with soap and water. What should she do next?

Procedure: Splinter

1. Wash the area vigorously to remove germs.
2. Use tweezers to remove surface splinters.
3. If a splinter is embedded in the skin, sterilize a needle by boiling it for 15 minutes, and use it to loosen the splinter. Slide the needle along the edge of the splinter to raise it to the skin's surface. Then use the tweezers to remove the splinter.
4. After removing the splinter, wash the area again.
5. If the splinter is lodged too deeply to remove it, have the victim see a doctor.
6. Look for signs of infection: swelling, tenderness, redness, throbbing, and pus.

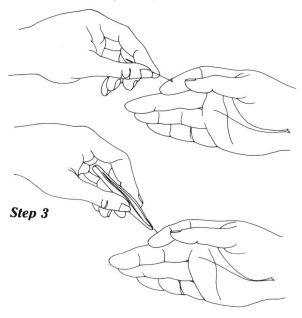

Step 3

Stroke

About strokes

Each year, over half a million adults suffer cardiovascular accidents, or strokes. More than half that number die. The victims who survive, however, are recovering with a reduced incidence of permanent damage.

Improved emergency and hospital care, new drugs, and advances in rehabilitation are among the reasons for recovery from stroke. Although the extent of the brain damage incurred at the time of the stroke determines the possibility of full recovery, the attitude of the victim and those around him greatly influences the outcome.

In some cases, tests can reveal the cause of the stroke, and delicate brain surgery or other treatment may prevent a second stroke.

When the blood supply to part of the brain becomes impaired, a stroke results. The brain area that doesn't receive its normal blood supply will no longer function in the usual manner. Anyone suffering from high blood pressure and hardening of the arteries is a potential stroke candidate. The signs and symptoms of a stroke depend on the area of the brain that is affected.

Signs and symptoms: Major stroke
1. Sudden headache.
2. Weakness, numbness, or paralysis down one side of the body.
3. Difficulty speaking or seeing.
4. Possible collapse and unconsciousness.
5. Difficulty breathing or swallowing.
6. Loss of bladder and bowel control.
7. Pupils unequal in size.
8. Convulsions.
9. Confusion.

Procedure: Major stroke
1. Maintain an open airway, and give artificial respiration, if necessary.
2. Loosen tight clothing; keep the victim at rest.
3. If the victim is unconscious, don't try to give him any fluids by mouth. Turn him on his side to allow secretions to drain from his mouth.
4. Slightly elevate the victim's head, neck, and shoulders, if possible.
5. Seek medical attention immediately.

Signs and symptoms: Minor stroke
1. Dizziness.
2. Headache.
3. Sudden memory impairment.
4. Weakness in an arm or leg.
5. Confusion.
6. Minor speech difficulty.

Procedure: Minor stroke
1. Protect the victim from falling.
2. Observe the victim for any further changes.
3. Seek medical help immediately.

Suicide Attempts

Ordinary, everyday depression usually passes after a brief period. Some people, however, suffer debilitating depressions, which may even be life-threatening. If a person becomes so disturbed by real or imaginary events that he threatens to take his own life, anyone trying to help must first reassure the potential victim while distracting him from his plan. At the first warning signs, people close to the potential victim should seek professional help.

A potential suicide victim may, on the other hand, be very secretive. He may not announce his plan, and he may hide harmful implements or drugs. In such cases, people trying to help will have to rely on their instincts, cautiously observe him, and offer concern and companionship.

Warning signals: Potential suicide

1. A direct threat of suicide with or without the means at hand.
2. Severe depression, acute anxiety, and prolonged grief.
3. Loss of appetite and insomnia.
4. Crying spells.
5. Heavy drinking or drug use.
6. Family history of suicide.
7. Giving away valuables.
8. Lack of interest in life over a long period of time.

Procedure: Potential suicide

1. Do not place yourself in danger. Make sure the scene is safe and the victim does not have a weapon.
2. Seek professional help for the victim.
3. Keep all harmful implements and drugs away from the victim.
4. Don't leave the victim alone.
5. Be a sympathetic listener, and encourage other friends and family members to do the same.
6. Take all threats seriously.

*Procedure:
When the victim has
a weapon or
suicide is imminent*
- *Remain calm. Have someone get medical help and call the police.*
- *Speak gently and don't argue with the victim.*
- *Don't try to force suicide implements or weapons from the victim.*
- *Ask the person if you can help or if he is hurt.*
- *Listen to the victim and let him know that you're paying attention.*
- *Don't make any sudden movements.*

Unconsciousness

Caution: Don't mistake unconsciousness for cardiac and respiratory failure.

Unconsciousness can be a difficult emergency to deal with because the causes are often not obvious. Among the possible causes of unconsciousness are head injury, diabetic coma, stroke, poisoning, shock, epilepsy, heart attack, fainting, and drug overdose.

Sign or symptom: Unconsciousness
The victim doesn't respond to attempts to awaken him.

Procedure: Unconsciousness
1. Establish that the victim is unconscious by trying to awaken him. In a loud voice, ask the victim if he is all right.
2. Have someone call an ambulance immediately.
3. Check the victim's airway and pulse, and give artificial respiration and CPR, if necessary. (See Artificial Respiration, pp. 20-21, and CPR, pp. 32-34.)
4. Loosen tight clothing.
5. Don't move the victim unless the victim's life is in jeopardy. If you must move him, move him "all in one piece". Do not bend his neck or back. (See Head, Neck, and Spine Injuries, pp. 27-30.)
6. Look for injuries and control any bleeding.
7. Don't give the victim liquids or solid food.
8. Keep the victim comfortably warm.
9. Don't place a pillow under the victim's head.
10. Check for a medical I.D. bracelet or card that indicates the victim's medical condition.
11. Don't leave the victim unattended.
12. If the victim wakes normally, try to keep the victim awake and ask him about possible reasons for his unconsciousness.

Check the ABC's
Follow the three-step procedure on pp. 6-7 to find out if the victim is breathing, and take the victim's pulse. When you can't feel a pulse, you know that the victim's heart has probably stopped.

Vomiting

Caution: Anytime a person who is unconscious or very weak vomits, turn the person onto his side so that the fluids drain out of his mouth and not down his throat or into his lungs.

Vomiting is a common physical disorder. When emotional upset, overeating, excessive intake of alcohol, minor food poisoning, or a viral intestinal infection is the cause of the vomiting, the victim usually feels better within 1 or 2 days. Vomiting that lasts longer requires medical attention.

Vomiting can also be a symptom of many serious illnesses such as appendicitis, bowel obstruction, black widow or brown recluse spider bite, poisonous snakebite, drug withdrawal, head injury, shock, heat exhaustion, food poisoning, hepatitis, and diabetic coma.

Warning signs and symptoms: Vomiting

Call a doctor immediately if the vomiting:
1. Lasts more than 1 or 2 days.
2. Is accompanied by severe abdominal pain.
3. Occurs with fever and abdominal pain.
4. Follows a recent head or abdominal injury.
5. Follows overexertion on a hot day.
6. Occurs with frequent diarrhea and severe abdominal cramps.
7. Contains blood or material that looks like coffee grounds.

Procedure: Vomiting without danger signs

1. Have the victim avoid solid foods.
2. Have the victim replace fluid loss by frequently sipping small amounts of water or flat ginger ale. Tea and both are also acceptable. Flat cola is acceptable if the victim does not have diarrhea.
3. If the victim cannot drink the liquids, let him suck on ice chips.
4. When the victim stops vomiting, first introduce bland foods such as dry toast, jello, and applesauce. Increase the amount of liquids.

Wounds

- *the wound is deep.*
- *the victim has not had a tetanus shot within 5 to 7 years.*
- *blood is spurting from the wound.*
- *bleeding persists despite efforts to control it.*
- *skin or tissue is ripped away.*
- *the victim received a puncture wound.*
- *the victim received an animal or human bite.*
- *a foreign object is embedded in the wound.*
- *the wound is on the face or on a body part where scar tissue will be noticeable after the wound heals.*
- *the wound is jagged or irregular.*

An injury that breaks the skin or the mucous membrane results in an open wound. With any type of open wound, primary concerns should be to:

1. Stop the bleeding.
2. Prevent infection.
3. Prevent or treat shock.
4. Seek medical attention, if necessary.

Open wounds: Abrasions

Scraping or "skinning" a knee or elbow results in an abrasion. Abrasions usually heal within a few days.

Procedure: Abrasions

1. Wash your hands before you wash the injured area with soap and water.
2. Cover the abrasion only if it's a large wound.
3. Don't use topical medication.
4. Watch for signs of infection that may appear after 1 or 2 days. (Signs of infection: pus, pain, redness, tenderness, a sensation of heat, and swelling.)
5. See a doctor if the wound is very large or if it becomes infected.

Open wounds: Cuts

A cut is a tear in the skin that also involves tissue under the skin surface. Incisions are smooth cuts, while lacerations are jagged or irregular cuts.

Procedure: Cuts

1. Wash your hands.
2. Wash the wound with soap and water.
3. Apply direct pressure to the wound to stop bleeding, if necessary.
4. Cover the wound with a sterile dressing that is larger than the wound.

Caution: Never remove an impaled object because the victim might bleed uncontrollably.

Open wounds: Puncture wounds

When David Grant leaned against a fence that had several nails sticking out of the wood he received three puncture wounds on his back. The wounds looked like small holes in his skin and bled very little.

A puncture wound occurs when a sharp object pierces layers of skin, underlying tissue, and possibly the organs in its path. Pins and nails often cause puncture wounds. Because puncture wounds often don't bleed freely and usually are deep and narrow, infection may very likely set in. Before treatment, a person should consider whether a joint, tendon, the skull, abdomen, or thoracic cavity has been affected by the wound. Someone with a puncture wound should also check to see whether the wound contains a foreign body.

Procedure: Puncture wounds

1. Wash your hands with soap and water.
2. Check to see if part of the object that caused the wound has remained in the wound.
3. Wash the wound with soap and water if the object isn't still embedded. If the object is still embedded, cover the wound around the object. Don't apply any pressure to the object.
4. Cover the wound with a sterile dressing.
5. Treat the victim for shock, if necessary.
6. Have the victim see a doctor unless the wound is minor and the victim has received a tetanus shot recently.

Closed wounds

In the case of a closed wound, the skin is unbroken. If the victim has been in an accident, however, he may have serious internal injuries despite not having an open wound. (See Bleeding, pp. 14-18, and Head, Neck, and Spine Injuries, pp. 27-30.)

Foreign body in a wound
• *Don't try to remove a foreign body embedded in a wound unless it comes out easily.*
• *Dress the wound with a ring pad instead, and see a doctor.*
• *Make a ring pad with a narrow bandage and padding such as a rolled up piece of cloth.*
• *After you make the ring pad:*
1. Clean the wound.
2. Place dry gauze over it.
3. Place the ring pad over the gauze.
4. Cover the pad.

Wrapping a joint wound

• A tight bandage will interfere with circulation and nerve function, and a loose one will do nothing.

• Don't overstretch elastic bandages or the bandage will be too tight.

• Never apply a wet gauze bandage because it will shrink when it dries and become too tight.

• Loosen bandages that become tight.

• Start a bandage from the inside of a limb, and finish it on the outside with a closure away from the body.

• Never start a bandage over a bone.

• Never put a bandage around a person's neck.

• Leave fingertips exposed when you bandage an arm or hand.

• Leave toes exposed when you bandage a foot or leg so you can check bandage tightness.

• Leave fingers exposed when you bandage a hand or wrist.

• Watch for swelling, discoloration, or cool skin around a bandage.

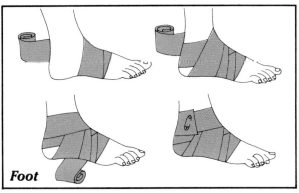

Foot

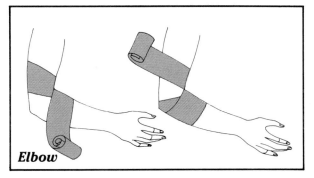

Elbow

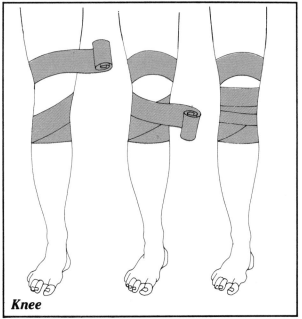

Knee

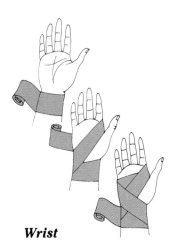

Wrist

Index